D0193825

Publication Data

Sarah Viola, *OTR/L, CDP, CDCS*
When Waves Rise – First edition.
Summary: "Education and practical strategies caregivers need to navigate difficult moments related to dementia." – Provided by publisher.
ISBN: 978-1-736814-50-5
[1. When Waves Rise – Non-Fiction] I. Title.

This book has been written with the published intent to provide accurate and authoritative information in regard to the subject matter included. While every reasonable precaution has been taken in preparation of this book the author and publisher expressly disclaim responsibility for any errors, omissions, or adverse effects arising from the use or application of the information contained inside. The techniques and suggestions are to be used at the reader's discretion and are not to be considered a substitute for professional medical care.

Graphic Designers Name: Angela Goehring, Simple Wolf Media, Ellendale ND

MEET THE FOUNDER AND AUTHOR

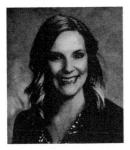

Sarah Viola, *OTR/L, CDP, CDCS*

Sarah Viola has been specializing in the care of those living with cognitive impairment, specifically dementia, for over ten years. Her love for those living with cognitive dysfunction began when she was in college and became extraordinarily strong while completing a fieldwork experience at the North Dakota State Hospital in Jamestown, ND.

She felt a strong pull to serve those she felt had a risk of "losing their voice," limiting their ability to live a life of their choosing as their disability progressed.

Throughout her career, Sarah has studied many models of dementia care. Through professional implementation, she realized there were specific skills that she was consistently teaching to care providers that helped them create a better quality of life for themselves and those in their care.

It was through this work that *Ever-Present Insight* came into existence. The logo for *Ever-Present Insight* is that of waves within helping hands. Sarah's personal goal is to help care partners learn vital skills in creating success for the person receiving care, yet give and receive grace throughout the journey. Just as waves and ripples in water ebb and flow, accepting changes in weather and debris yet calming once again in the right conditions, we can provide this type of grace to ourselves and our loved ones while navigating through living with dementia. We must always remember the ever-present nature of individuals' spirits that makes them unique and guides care as we partner with them on the journey.

As you read, please remember these mottos from Sarah:

1. "You are the key to unlocking your loved one's potential, the medication they need daily."

2. "If you are trying, you are succeeding; perfection is not possible."

TABLE OF CONTENTS

1) Dedication   page 1
2) Foreword by Naomi Evans M.S. CCC-SLP   page 2
3) Introduction   page 3
4) Foundational Insights
    a. The Brain   page 6
    b. Communication   page 12
    c. The Person   page 16

5) Insight for Specific Moments   page 24

    a. The Initial Moment   page 26

    b. A Routine Moment   page 30

    c. Anticipate the Moment   page 34

    d. Mold the Moment   page 42

    e. Embrace the Moment   page 48

    f. Study the Moment   page 52

    g. Save the Moment   page 62

    h. Shift the Moment   page 70

    i. Confirm the Moment   page 76

    j. Remember the Moment   page 82

6) References   page 90
7) Appendix A: Expressive Behaviors   page 92
8) Appendix B: Recommended Resources   page 108

(A note: Throughout this text, dementia and cognitive impairment or cognitive dysfunction will be used synonymously.)

DEDICATION

This training opportunity is dedicated to my grandmother, a woman who fully lived yet died with dementia.

A woman who refueled my passion for serving those living with dementia after feeling helpless watching individuals and families struggle for years navigating this disease.

A woman who proved to me that as I used my heart, skill, and passion for helping her live her life with dementia, my attempts were not in vain.

A woman who taught me that there will be heartache in life, but that through faith, we can choose to keep living and find joy despite those heartaches.

FOREWORD

Many years ago, when I was fresh out of graduate school, I walked into my new place of employment, a nursing home. I began my clinical fellowship year as a speech-language pathologist, helping some of our most vulnerable with their swallowing functions, cognitive functions, voice production, and speech and language skills. I had big aspirations, as does every student just finishing college. My expectations were high. When I walked into this nursing home, I could not believe my eyes. I saw people slumped in wheelchairs, just sitting there. The staff members appeared to be entirely too busy to handle anything except the necessary. I could feel the stress and tension in the building. There was so much to do, yet so little time—except for those residents; they did not have much of anything to do. They had all the time in the world to sit and stare. My heart broke and still does when I think back on that day.

As of 2016, the CDC reports that nearly 50 percent of residents living in nursing homes have dementia. The Alzheimer's Association says that almost six million Americans suffer from dementia, and this number will grow exponentially to nearly fourteen million by midcentury.

Skilled care for those living with dementia in this country has improved since the days of my naïve venture to save the world. However, I do believe we, as a nation, still have a long way to go. Did you notice I previously wrote that six million Americans "suffer" from dementia? That is true, right? We believe that someone diagnosed with any form of dementia will suffer, and their loved ones are sure to suffer too. But hear me out. There might be another way.

After spending my workdays in multiple skilled nursing facilities day in and day out, my focus evolved. I was fortunate to be mentored by a speech-language pathologist who had a great perspective on dementia and caring for those living with dementia. Her enthusiasm, humor, and the day-to-day joy she brought to each resident she encountered were evident and contagious. Her theory was, "Why merely survive if we can instead help these folks thrive?!" Unbeknownst to me at the time, that philosophy would shape so much of my life and my family's life. It would be the beginning of an adventure to help others shift their thinking regarding dementia and other conditions traditionally viewed in a negative light, a shift from negative thoughts to positive thoughts. A necessary shift to help those living with this disease maintain purpose, pleasure, and joy. So please read on! Learn from one of the best, my sister, Sarah Viola, and help us shift the focus of dementia care from merely surviving to THRIVING!

Naomi Evans, M.S. CCC-SLP

INTRODUCTION

Listen closely to people who have cared for or who are currently caring for a person living with dementia or other cognitive impairments. While listening, whether it is to a hired care partner or a family member, you may hear a mixture of the thoughts below.

- Marion always wants to "go home" even though she is already at her home.
- Bob will not take his pills because he thinks they are poison.
- Bonnie will not take her pills because she believes "the orange one" gives her a headache.
- Julie has stopped getting dressed in the morning and only wants to wear her pajamas.
- Mike has stopped attending previously enjoyed outings and engagements.
- Bernice is losing weight; she tells me she is eating, but I do not see any evidence.
- Dennis refuses to attend meals within his care community.
- Delores becomes increasingly agitated in the late afternoon and appears frustrated, anxious, and angry at times.
- Vern loses his temper quickly over small things.
- Martha refuses to bathe, which is odd because she has always been so attuned to her appearance.
- Andy wakes up and wanders during overnight hours.
- Mary wakes up and talks about the people in her room.
- Francis gets anxious and calls me obsessively, asking the same questions repeatedly.
- William calls me angry almost daily because "I forgot something" or "Messed something up."
- Rose gets upset, telling me to leave each time I come over to help her.

Do these moments sound familiar? As a care partner for someone living with cognitive impairment, you may have encountered one or more of the situations described above. That list is not exhaustive, of course, and you may have experienced other difficult moments not described. The purpose of this material is to assist you, the care partner, in managing moments like these with confidence.

Suppose we help you recognize cognitive impairment, understand why it may be happening, and maintain hope that positive outcomes are possible. With that belief in mind, modification of thinking and actions can then create these positive outcomes. It starts with you, the care partner. As Dr. Seuss (1971) once wrote, "Unless someone like you cares a whole awful lot, nothing is going to get better. It's not."

In the sections that follow, we will first review foundational principles and then dive into specific moments, giving you tools for creating positive outcomes.

FOUNDATIONAL INSIGHTS

The following section will provide brief foundational knowledge. The topics included are intended to help you identify essential knowledge that will help you understand the ten *Insights for Specific Moments* that follow. The explanation and breakdown of the content are designed to be brief and simplified.

PART 1:

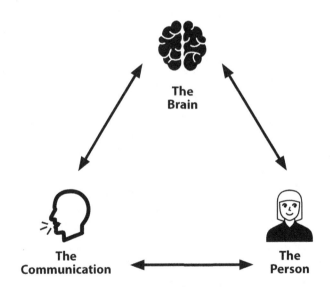

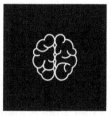

INSIGHT ABOUT THE BRAIN

"If the human brain were so simple that we could understand it, we would be so simple that we couldn't."

– Emerson M Pugh

If we want to learn more about dementia and what people are experiencing when they live with dementia, there is no more appropriate place to start than the brain.

The brain and body's relationship is like a hard drive to a computer. Our brain determines everything we think, say, or do throughout the day. It controls our bodies in both conscious and unconscious ways. The reason physicians do brain scans to check for activity to prove life or death is that our brains drive every process in our bodies, both inward and outward. The medical community is still working to more fully understand the incredible organ that is the brain.

When the brain functions in an unimpaired capacity, we call that "intact cognition." If an impairment impacts centers of the brain, we call that either major or minor neurocognitive disorder or delirium. Any form of dementia falls under this neurocognitive disorder umbrella. Cognitive impairment that creates dementia does not have to be memory or loss of words, common in Alzheimer's-type dementia. Other types of dementia include, but are not limited to, frontotemporal dementia, dementia with Lewy bodies, Parkinson's-type dementia, vascular dementia, and alcohol or substance-induced dementia. These varying types of dementias all have indicative signs and symptoms due to the different locations of impairment in the brain. The effect of brain loss or atrophy can be complicated. The signs and symptoms of each impairment, along with the severity, will reflect where the impairment is in the brain and to what extent.

Brain Functions

To help understand the types of dementia better, let us dive a little deeper into how the brain works. The brain has many centers that house different functions, and there are pathways between these centers that communicate with each other. If an outward impairment is present, the dysfunction may be in one of the centers that control that function or in the pathways between the centers. The center of the brain housing the function and the pathway to keep the centers communicating must be working correctly to execute a desired behavior or action.

Examples of brain functions include (not a comprehensive list):

- Planning (thinking about the steps of activity to obtain goals – visualizing what is needed)

  i.e., looking at your GPS to plan where you will stop for gas on a road trip, so you don't run out.

- Initiation of Action (taking action to achieve a goal – taking the first step)

  i.e., deciding to get up and walk over to the faucet for a drink since you are thirsty.

- Self-Control (regulating oneself regarding external stimuli)

  i.e., finding yourself in a situation making you angry and breathing deep to allow yourself to calm down before reacting.

- Emotional Regulation (responding to the environment with appropriate emotions)

  i.e., laughing when something is funny, crying when you are sad, responding in a controlled fashion with your emotions.

- Problem-Solving (recognize the problem, devise a solution, implement a solution, analyze the solution)

  i.e., running out of toothpaste, knowing you are out, and going to the store to get more rather than brushing your teeth without any toothpaste.

- Attention (types: sustained, switching, divided, selective)

  i.e., listening to a lecture

  i.e., eating, then stopping to chat with a partner, then going back to eating

  i.e., eating while listening to music

  i.e., listening to a lecture and not attending to the background noises you hear around you.

- Abstract Thinking (using concepts to understand generalizations; thinking and understanding the unseen)

  i.e., the ability to understand what someone is asking you to do when asking you a vague or open-ended question.

- Visual/Spatial Perception – (recognizing objects, their location, and orientation in space)

  i.e., understanding what you are looking at and using this information or navigating through a tight maze without bumping into the walls.

- Sequencing (directing oneself through the correct steps to accomplish a task in the right order)

  i.e., knowing you have to take off your clothes first to wash up, dry off, and then re-dress.

- Memory (types: short-term, working, long-term, and procedural)

  i.e., taking in new information to remember it immediately

  i.e., using new information, such as navigating a new cell phone

  i.e., remembering information from a past time period

  i.e., using old memories or routines to be able to accomplish a task.

- Language (expressive and receptive)

  i.e., sending a message to a friend via verbal/nonverbal communication

  i.e., taking in and understanding information/messages sent by another person.

As you can see from this list and examples, these processes are complex, and the complexity does not end here. Within the brain, there are also workers and traffic controllers. The workers perform the brain's functions. Before the workers can perform any function, the traffic controllers have to tell them when and how to perform. The traffic controllers essentially tell the workers to start the car and drive. Think about the traffic controllers as stoplights: when they give you the green light, you go or do, and when they give you a red light, you stop. They may even provide a yellow light at times, which tells you to think through a situation before acting.

These functions, including the workers and traffic controllers, are contained in various lobes of the brain. Brain lobes each house the different cognitive functions described above. Both workers and traffic controllers are housed in multiple lobes of the brain; however, a majority of traffic controllers are housed in the frontal lobe. As discussed earlier, the brain's lobes and centers are important to maintain function. But we need to remember that the pathways between these lobes are equally important when considering proper functionality and the effects of impairment.

Brain Lobes

Each of the lobes, or centers of the brain, primarily hold certain functions. However, it is not as straightforward as it sounds. Because our human brain is so complex, some functions are housed throughout a few different lobes of the brain, each location holding a piece of the function and pathways connecting the whole circuit. The following list describes the primary functions housed in the varying lobes to provide you a road map of function (not a comprehensive list):

- Frontal Lobe
  Emotional Regulation, Planning, Reasoning, Problem-Solving, Judgment, Inhibition of Behavior, Attention, Expressive Language

- Parietal Lobe
  Integration of Sensory Information (touch, taste, pain), Visual and Spatial Perception

- Temporal Lobe
  Memory, Hearing, Receptive Language, Organizing, and Sequencing (thinking skills)

- Occipital Lobe
  Visual Processing (depth perception, distance/location of objects in the environment)

- Cerebellum
  Coordination, Balance, Equilibrium

- Brain Stem
  Breathing, Heart Rate, Swallowing, Reflexes, Control of Autonomic Functions, Sleep, Sense of Balance

Any disruption in a lobe or in the pathways connecting one lobe to another may cause impairment. The complexity that exists in our human brain is extraordinary and difficult to understand. Thus, rather than knowing all the brain functions, we, as care partners, need to put ourselves in our loved one's shoes so we can modify and adapt to identified needs in each moment. Learning the brain's basics can help us understand the complexity and vast array of malfunctions a brain can have. This knowledge helps us understand and empathize with people who are living with cognitive impairment. Understanding and empathizing then allow us to modify moments to meet the needs of our loved ones appropriately.

An impaired brain will become more rigid and unable to adapt to the outside world, worsening throughout the disease process. A cognitively intact brain will have the flexibility to modify and adjust to a loved one or care recipient.

To summarize brain functions and lobes:

1. There are many different cognitive processes in your brain.
2. These cognitive processes work together to make up the function of the whole brain.
3. Any time one or more brain areas or pathways connecting these areas are impaired, the result could be described as dementia.
4. Cognitive dysfunction is real and creates impairment that we will never fully understand. Due to this, we need to be gracious, merciful, and empathetic toward others when we encounter people living with impairment.

Dementia Stages or Levels

Try not to stress all this medical knowledge about the brain. Instead, think about it therapeutically. The extent of cognitive impairment can be better understood through the use of stages or levels. Learning these cognitive stages or levels can provide a framework for care partners to understand better the abilities and needs of the person living with impairment.

In occupational therapy, a scale called the Allen Cognitive Levels is utilized to help outline varying stages. The Allen Cognitive Levels identify remaining abilities at each stage to help care partners understand how best to support their loved ones and know what level of independence is safe in daily living.

The Allen Cognitive Levels range from level six (intact cognition) to level one (end-stage dementia). Level five defines mild cognitive impairment, and level four is considered an early stage of dementia. Level three and level two are both stages of dementia, with the severity of impairment worsening as the numbers descend. Each level has stepwise modes to add greater detail to the remaining abilities individuals possess despite their dementia diagnosis. Understanding these strengths and weaknesses helps care partners provide the appropriate support to optimize their loved ones' function.

Additionally, being aware of these strengths and weaknesses helps professionals and care partners structure the environment and living arrangements to provide appropriate safety measures. Often care partners are thinking, "I'm not sure what is safe or possible for my loved one." These levels help establish a foundation in which care partners can feel confident, knowing they are providing the right level of assistance and making the necessary modifications to ensure safety and success for their loved ones each day.

Cognitive levels are somewhat lengthy to learn; thus, reaching out to skilled professionals is the most effective way for a care partner to obtain the necessary information. Therapy staff, specifically occupational therapists, are uniquely trained to assess individuals and determine which level or stage an individual is functioning within concerning cognitive impairment. Throughout this assessment, therapists can lay out a foundation for care partners to provide detailed guidance so they know how to adapt to their loved ones' needs. Suppose the environmental factors (care partner and environment) adapt to support the defined limitations. In that case, individuals with dementia can still complete skills and tasks to the best of their abilities, rather than having tasks taken away when they begin to struggle with parts.

Here is an example of what a therapist may do for clients and their care partners. If an individual with impairment is having difficulty getting dressed, a trained occupational therapist can determine which cognitive skill is impaired, leading to this difficulty. The therapist will then provide cues to compensate for the deficit area. Cues might include verbal directions for each step of the task or merely assisting with the task's initiation. Grading a task is a unique skill of therapists, and the purpose is to make the task more or less complicated through the type and number of external supports used. Therapists can help care partners determine what is and is not working, and educate them on how they can adapt daily to create success.

As we continue, we will explore specific moments and insights related to these moments. We will reference the cognitive functions reviewed previously and consider which function is impaired and how we might compensate for that impairment. These adaptations, modifications, and cues all center around two crucial things: communication and personal interaction.

The Brain Takeaways:

- The brain is so complex, and any impairment of a particular area or the pathway between specific areas can create dysfunction. The impairments explain why your loved one may be acting a certain way; however, the person cannot change his or her behavior due to these real deficits.

- Seek support and assistance from skilled professionals to help you better understand your loved one's brain. This understanding will allow you to experience positive outcomes through specialized, customized interventions designed for positive results.

PART 2

INSIGHT ABOUT COMMUNICATION

"We see that every external motion, act, gesture, whether voluntary or mechanical, organic or mental, is produced by internal feeling or emotion, will or volition, and thought of mind."

– Helena Blavatsky

Bernice is feeling restless. She gets up from the table and begins hurriedly walking away. Her care partner knows Bernice is only halfway done with her meal and has a goal of telling Bernice that she needs to sit back down to finish her meal so that she can feel full and comfortable.

The care partner approaches Bernice with her arms in a position that visually tells Bernice to stop walking and says, "Bernice, you need to sit down. You aren't finished with your meal, and you love meatloaf."

Bernice is startled by the care partner and pushes past her forcefully. Bernice continues to walk away from her meal with even more vigor than before.

The care partner's communication made Bernice defensive. Even though the intent was helpful and not harmful, the message Bernice received did not match the care partner's intention. What happened? Where was the disconnect that created this adverse outcome?

Communication is a large part of how we interact with our world. Communication is the way we take in information and send information to others around us. With both verbal and nonverbal strategies, we communicate our needs and wants and enjoy relationships with others. If you have ever had a conflict in a relationship or business encounter, you may have heard, "There was a communication breakdown." As we interact with individuals with cognitive impairment, the need for added attention to communication grows. Traditional forms of communication—spoken words—become distorted for someone with an impairment. Such individuals begin to rely on nonverbal communication. Therefore, as their communication partners, we also need to rely on nonverbal forms to match our loved ones' current strengths.

Each person uses different vocal characteristics to relay intent to another person. Our verbal messages are affected by tone, stress, pitch, volume, intonation, and speed. Also, body language, posture, gestures, and facial expressions contribute to the message we convey. These nonverbal signals play a significant role in the actual message we send. The spoken words we use are just a small part of how we deliver our message. Statistics show us that 55 percent of our message comes from our body language, 38 percent comes from tone of voice, and only 7 percent of the message is delivered through the actual words we use (Mehrabian, 2007).

When communicating with a person who has dementia, there is one rule: if there is a communication breakdown, YOU must change or modify your message to match your communication partner's ability to receive the message. You must adjust body language, intonation, gestures, and words to match your loved one's ability to comprehend the message. Changing your delivery will ensure your intended message is received accurately.

The following are a few tips to modify your verbal communication to assist the receiver in understanding:

- Use short and simple phrases and words
- Use everyday language from the person's past
- Repeat key words or phrases that you know resonated well, to prevent the person from forgetting the message
- Use the person's name
- Use concrete words and language
- Use suggestions rather than questions
- Adjust wording or phrases before repeating yourself if your message did not resonate.

To modify your nonverbal communication to assist the receiver in better understanding:

- Smile
- Gain and maintain eye contact
- Highlight key words in your phrase through your intonation
- Slow your rate of speech
- Pause or wait for a response
- Relax your face and body by taking a few deep breaths
- Uncross your arms
- Position your body in a nonthreatening way
- Communicate at eye level
- Sit down to provide visual representation that you are not in a hurry
- Offer a gentle touch
- Use gestures to help increase understanding
- Listen with your whole face and body
- Eliminate distractions to add focus for you and your communication partner
- Use a mirror to help you visually see what your nonverbals are communicating before communicating with your partner.

Communication is a foundational piece that will be discussed throughout each of the ten moments in this book. The first step in communication is the art of listening. Too often, care partners are consumed with "What will I say next?" or "How can I phrase this so it resonates?" especially as communication becomes more and more distorted or challenging. Find a way to minimize your fear response in communication so that you can focus on listening, allowing your communication to flow naturally.

Your rate of speech needs to slow significantly as cognition worsens. Slowing your communication style will allow you time to think on your feet after hearing, listening, and understanding your loved one. This slow rate also gives your loved one the best chance of comprehending your intended message. Remember, you cannot change how your loved one's brain will receive/understand your message, but you can change how your message is delivered. Modify your delivery to match your loved one's ability to comprehend.

As you slow the rate of the communication exchange, empathy is critical. You must convey empathy in your response; match your loved one's emotional state through your response. Throughout the disease process, communication becomes an emotionally driven process that is needs-based rather than pleasurable. Thus, we need to slow down to detect what emotions or needs are present for our loved ones. Helena Blavatsky states, "We see that every external motion, act, gesture, whether voluntary or mechanical, organic or mental, is produced by internal feeling or emotion, will or volition, and thought of mind" (Brainy Quotes, 2020). We must maintain this belief as cognition fades so that we never lose sight of the person within.

Communication Takeaways:

- If the message your loved one receives/understands is the same as the message you sent/intended, there is no communication breakdown. However, if the received message does not equal the intended message, there is a communication breakdown.

- We cannot change how our loved one can process/receive the message, so we must change the way our message is delivered.

- Deliver your intended message in such a way as to match your loved one's ability to receive the message. YOU manage the modification of your communication in the moment.

PART 3
INSIGHT ABOUT THE PERSON

Person-centered care is "a partnership aimed towards improving and maintaining a person's quality of care by recognizing and meeting the human needs of comfort, attachment, inclusion, identity, occupation and love."

– Thomas Kitwood

Education about cognitive impairment and good dementia care is person-centered care, keeping the person as the focal point of what we do, never losing sight of him or her. As our loved one changes, shifts, and adapts to a new normal, a life with cognitive impairment, we need to keep him or her as our focus. Dr. Al Power stated a new definition for dementia. He said, "Dementia is simply a shift in the way a person experiences the world" (Power, 2010). Following this excellent definition, Power explains that due to this shift in how a person experiences the world, we must also shift to create success.

As you and your loved one change together, be cautious not to lose sight of who the person is. Some types of cognitive impairment have the potential to alter your loved one's personality or mood. As the person living with intact cognition, you want to uphold who your loved one was before diagnosis and bring this forth into a new normal. Bridging this gap is a key to minimizing or even preventing difficult moments in the coming days. To bridge the gap, we first need to understand our loved one's intricacies.

16

Person-Centered Care

Person-centered care began with a professor, Tom Kitwood. His work helped reshape a person's view of individuals living with dementia and what they may be going through each day. He studied individuals who were living with both reversible and irreversible dementia. Through his study, he developed a perspective of great importance that we can all learn from today.

Professor Kitwood teaches that an individual has six psychological needs: comfort, attachment, inclusion, identity, occupation, and love (1997). As an occupational therapist specializing in the care of those living with dementia, I've found these six psychological needs to be a key component to understanding an individual living with dementia and what we, as outsiders, might be seeing as moments arise. These psychological needs greatly influence a person's behavior, and as we learned, dementia impacts our complex brain function. Therefore, we need to adjust ourselves psychologically, keeping our loved ones at the focus and appreciating all their intricacies.

People are complex creatures. We are all wired in different ways that add diversity and uniqueness to this world. This foundation of "who we are" is key to our preferences. Understanding oneself and the people around us in a more precise capacity can help us be therapeutic in our relationships with others and be improved through emotional intelligence. This understanding and how we use it to impact those around us is a significant key to working with a loved one living with dementia. (Please note: as mentioned early in this text, in this learning material, you will read about both cognitive impairment and dementia. Dementia is a type of cognitive impairment, and these words may be used interchangeably.)

Emotional Intelligence & Therapeutic Use of Self

Emotional intelligence is the capacity to understand yourself and those around you (Goleman, 2011). Emotional intelligence helps us use ourselves therapeutically for the benefit of our loved ones. If we are willing to study ourselves, every person can be quite effective at working with those living with dementia.

If you can read the person, read yourself, and respond in a way that adjusts to that person and situation, you will be most effective. For example:

You walk into a room. A man with dementia is sitting with his arms crossed and has restless legs. You notice that when you enter, he clams up even more. You know he is a retired physician who has always received the utmost respect from people in his presence. You also understand that he has insight into his impairment but is having trouble accepting the new diagnosis. You know that he has always been witty and sarcastic, and this humor is a way to break the ice.

What do you know about yourself? You know that you are outgoing, and your voice can be loud and intrusive. You know that standing over a person when he is seated presents itself as authoritative. You know that you need to shift your natural tendencies to meet/match this person's needs to build his trust so you can accomplish the goal at hand.

1. You take a deep breath to calm yourself, your speech rate, and your nonverbal message before beginning.
2. You approach with a humble handshake and greeting that shows respect as this gentleman has come to expect in years past. "Good afternoon, Dr. Strange." (This helps him uncross his arms so that he can begin to calm down.)
3. You ask if you can sit down beside him.
4. You sit after being instructed to (he directs the situation, not you).
5. You crack a joke about his favorite football team to lighten the mood.
6. You then begin a conversation about his interests and continue this conversation for approximately five minutes.

You notice that his shoulders have relaxed, his legs stop jittering, and his facial expressions are now calm and happy as you joke back and forth. Now you can try to switch gears gently into a conversation that will flow into your goal, always remembering to let him direct so as to preserve his sense of self.

According to Pryor Learning Solutions, a person needs to be personally and socially competent to have high emotional intelligence. Emotional intelligence is not something we are born with but rather is a skill we cultivate, nurture, and grow throughout our lifetime. Most people think having high emotional intelligence is about what you know. However, that is not the case. Emotional intelligence is about how well people can use and integrate intelligence and skills to affect the world around them. It is about understanding yourself and your traits and being able to use them effectively (Pryor Learning Solutions, 2018, p. 3). In the world of occupational therapy, we call this "therapeutic use of self," meaning each person can understand themselves and use themselves therapeutically to maximize their positive impact when working with others.

Understanding oneself, or emotional intelligence, can be looked at from two different lenses—being personally aware and able to manage oneself and being socially conscious and able to control oneself in social situations (Pryor Learning Solutions, 2018, p. 3). These two lenses of emotional intelligence become more evident as we build self-awareness. We build self-awareness by studying ourselves, studying situations we encounter, analyzing how we react or respond, and creating accurate perceptions.

After accurately perceiving ourselves, which is the first lens we look through, a person must manage his or her personal traits in dynamic situations, taking numerous years of trial and error or study to develop. You will experience ever-changing growth as you reflect and become more personally aware. Constant change can make us feel a lack of confidence in our abilities as we attempt to improve our emotional intelligence, and confidence is necessary to help with the ability to adapt in social situations as we build our self-awareness (Pryor Learning Solutions, 2018, p. 3).

So what do we do as we grow and lack the confidence needed to feel successful? Develop a belief of "trying is succeeding!" This can help you feel confident and make a conscious effort to learn, grow, and adapt. When learning through your experiences with a loved one who has dementia, this may feel quite daunting at times because each experience may not be pleasant. You may leave some interactions feeling like "I messed that one up." However, remember, you are trying, and because of that, you are succeeding.

Another great reminder comes from the book of Romans 5:3–4, "Not only so, but we also glory in our suffering, because we know that suffering produces perseverance; perseverance, character; and character, hope." Suffering can mean many things to many people. For our purposes, let's look at it in the context of meaning "going through something challenging" as we adopt this lens of "trying is succeeding." Then as we go through this suffering, we can be confident that we will persevere. It will build our character, which will provide the hope we need to continue learning and growing. Learning from our experiences is a key to creating this self-awareness.

Therefore, to succeed at personal growth and self-awareness, we need to take a step back, park our emotions, and accurately reflect on experiences to learn from them. Understanding who we are and how we tend to respond allows us to therapeutically use ourselves better in future situations when working with a loved one with dementia. You may be thinking, "I already have this figured out; I don't need to learn much more," and maybe you do. Nevertheless, it is critical to learn from our experiences to care for a loved one with dementia effectively.

As a care partner, you will experience both new and familiar situations, but you will do so through a different lens. It is this paradigm shift in our thinking that creates success. There will be trial and error, but it is through moments of error that we learn to use our therapeutic selves most effectively. Each time you experience a successful moment, it will fuel more hope for moments to come.

Social awareness is the second lens into understanding oneself. Social awareness refers to how well we can read other people's emotional states and how well we can understand other's complexities. Being able to demonstrate true empathy is a demonstration of good social awareness. As individuals, we are just one of two factors needed for a relationship, and as a part of the relationship, we have the power to influence. Situations can be difficult or easy depending on how well we align with the other individual with whom we are in a relationship. We must be able to manage situations, whether difficult or easy, and cooperate. To summarize this lens, Daniel Goleman states that emotional intelligence is "the capacity for recognizing our feelings and those of others, for motivating ourselves, and for managing emotions well in ourselves and our relationships" (Pryor Learning Solutions, 2018, p. 3).

As previously noted, emotional intelligence is key to reading and responding well, both personally and socially, in various situations throughout life. Emotional intelligence becomes of even greater importance if one of the individuals is living with cognitive impairment. The ability to "read and respond" (using logic and reasoning) rather than "read and react" (using our gut reaction or impulsive responses) has the potential to unlock success for the individual living with dementia. On the flip side, a lack of emotional intelligence can create difficult moments for the individual and the relationship. Care partners are the key to helping unlock a loved one's full potential day in and day out. We are the medications our loved ones need to take that can allow each day to flow with ease.

Personality Traits

To help you achieve emotional intelligence as described above, Pryor Learning Solutions describes a few personality styles that can provide insight. (Please note there are many different educational opportunities related to personality types, and you are encouraged to explore others to further your learning. These are easily understood and relate well to our education in this writing; thus, they are the traits we are using here.)

Common personality traits include extroverts, introverts, thinkers, and feelers. These four categories are not exclusive, meaning a person does not merely function within one category or trait. People can operate within each category (Pryor Learning Solutions, 2018, p. 5). As we review these personality traits, the key is to recognize where you and your loved one function primarily so you can adapt to these varying styles. Please keep the goal of building self-awareness front of mind; this self-awareness will be critical later when we study the top ten insights.

Extrovert characteristics (Pryor Learning Solutions, 2018, p. 6):
- Focused on people and the environment; socially driven
- Enjoy being a part of a team
- Talk things through to process them; "think out loud"

- May lose focus more quickly if a topic is long-winded
- Prefer verbal communication to written communication
- Are perceived as poor listeners
- Want action in experiences
- Talk too much or say things impulsively.

Introvert characteristics (Pryor Learning Solutions, 2018, p. 6):
- Focused on their inner world
- May be quieter in social situations or perceived this way
- Want work that is "head"-focused, thinking-focused
- Think before they act, which may be perceived as taking too long to make a decision
- Are perceived as good listeners
- Will shut down or change their thought process if forced to provide solutions/answers before they are ready
- Provide well-thought-out responses
- Like to write things down if they want to remember or process the information again later
- May talk more if interested or motivated by the subject

Thinker characteristics (Pryor Learning Solutions, 2018, p. 7):
- Enjoy facts and figures
- Make decisions through analysis and logical outcomes
- Excel in analytics
- Tend to view things as absolute, "all or none."
- Feel more comfortable with things in writing
- Define "rapport" with others as thinking similarly
- Fair to others; however, people are an afterthought
- Direct and to the point; do not elaborate with stories.

Feeler characteristics (Pryor Learning Solutions, 2018, p. 8):
- People are the forethought; prefer relationships and "rapport"
- May take things personally or overanalyze social interactions
- Want their feelings and the feelings of others to be recognized
- Can carry a grudge if feelings are hurt
- Are tactful

- Are sympathetic and empathetic
- Make decisions based on what is most important to the people involved, not necessarily logic
- Bring emotion into subjects, even if the issue is only facts and figures
- Share stories to validate thoughts and feelings when conversing with others.

Before you think, "What does this have to do with me learning about dementia and my loved one?", the intent of learning about extroverts, introverts, thinkers, and feelers is to help provide you with a foundation you can build from to become more self and socially aware. This self- and social awareness will develop your emotional intelligence. Emotional intelligence will be your best friend when it comes to therapeutically using yourself when working with your loved one living with cognitive impairment.

You have probably heard the phrase, "This is not about you." In the case of working with a loved one living with dementia, this has never been truer. It is not about you, even though you will go through a tremendous amount of change in the future, and at times this change may feel like too much. However, understanding yourself, reading your loved one, joining the person's reality, and matching your well-thought-out responses to his or her needs, will be the key to making each day successful.

The Person Takeaways:

- Personal interaction is a two-way street, and it encompasses every situation we have if we are with another human being. Whether you are having a conversation in passing or helping a person complete a task, you are in the middle of personal interaction. We need to caution ourselves never to lose sight of the personal interaction that is taking place.

- As we begin to care for another person, it may feel at times that we have a "checklist" of duties to complete with/for the individual. Fight this urge to check off your list and instead preserve the personal interaction that takes place as you assist the person with each item.

- Be therapeutic in using yourself, and remember your own characteristics as you work with your loved one.

- Also remember the other person's characteristics, the things that make the person unique. These characteristics should be your focus and guide throughout these interactions.

- Who are you as a person, and what are your preferences during an interaction? How do you come across from another's perspective? Practice modifying or adapting your interaction to suit varying individual needs you encounter.

- Who is the person you are working with, and what are his or her preferences during an interaction? How does the person come across from your perspective? Is it pleasant or unpleasant in your eyes? (Ask this of yourself to become more aware of your natural "reactions" to this person, not as a judgment call.)

- How can you use a grace-filled lens in daily interactions to perceive good, even when that is not what it looks like from the outside?

INSIGHTS FOR SPECIFIC MOMENTS

The following section will provide practical tips for care partners to support their loved ones living with dementia. Following each Insight, there will be journal pages to allow you to journal experiences, write questions or comments related to the reading, or share joyful moments to help maintain focus on the person in your care who is *Ever-Present*.

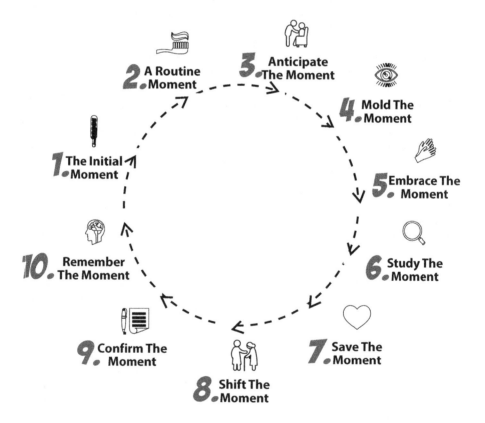

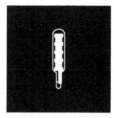

THE INITIAL MOMENT

I entered our living room, and my wife was sitting in her chair. All the lights were on, and there was music playing. I had had an exciting moment that I wanted to share with her. I approached her quickly, speaking rapidly in a bit of a loud voice. I began to describe why I was excited. As I approached, I noticed my wife's mood shift. She began to frown and turned away from me. I wondered why my excitement was not important to her. Why wasn't she happy for me?

What happened during this moment? My wife had known me for years and knew I was always an excitable person. Why was she caught off guard this time? But thinking about it more, I realized this type of moment had become more frequent.

Let us rewind a bit to analyze this couple's interaction. The care partner's excitement and speed of relation caused his wife to shut down. The care partner is confused and feels blown off. These moments that feel abnormal or unpredictable are a good indicator that you will need to start adjusting your delivery.

For your loved one, the ability to process sources of sensory information in the environment can change as cognitive impairment progresses. The ability to respond rationally or logically also changes because the brain does not send the signals through the proper channels, and thus a more "reactionary" response is typically seen. The limbic brain (not-conscious part, instinct brain) kicks in. If the information is not sent through to the cortex (the conscious center, thinking/

logical/reasoning brain), that reaction is noted because the whole brain has not had a chance to control the behavior. If a person has cognitive impairment, we must adjust how we begin interacting with our loved one as a care partner.

It is crucial that we "take the temperature" of each scenario before beginning interaction. What happened in the hours before the situation? How are your loved one's mood, demeanor, body language, facial expressions? What are the person's nonverbal messages telling you? Is the environment loud and distracting (overstimulating), or is it quiet and calm (under-stimulating)? Is the lighting adequate? Does your loved one see you approaching, and has the person had a chance to understand and accept the coming interaction? What is your loved one's personality—introverted, extroverted, thinker, or feeler—and how can you match or complement this in the exchange?

Taking the temperature of the scenario allows you to kick on your emotional intelligence and adjust to meet your loved one's temperature. This strategy shows an understanding of your loved one as a person and validates his or her emotions right from the start. You are the key that unlocks your loved one's potential in the upcoming interaction!

As discussed in the communication section, empathy is a crucial component to taking the temperature of the room and matching your temperature to your loved one. Pryor Learning Solutions states that empathy is "The capacity to share another person's position and emotions" (2018, p. 23). The ability to control your own emotions and actions is necessary when working with a person living with dementia.

The scenario above might have evolved differently if the care partner had been able to see that his wife would be overwhelmed by such a fast, excited approach. Instead, matching his emotional temperature to her emotional temperature and abilities would have allowed her to receive his intended message. Learning to listen without communicating, and listening with your eyes upon first interaction, *then* with your ears, is crucial. Each exchange will be set up for success if this is how the initial moments unfold.

The Initial Moment Takeaways:

- Take the room temperature.
- Analyze your loved one's emotional state.
- Consider the environment and surroundings to adapt your approach to match your loved one's ability to receive your upcoming message.

27

My thoughts:

_____

_____

_____

_____

_____

_____

_____

_____

_____

_____

_____

_____

_____

_____

_____

_____

_____

_____

_____

_____

_____

_____

_____

_____

_____

_____

_____

_____

_____

_____

_____

_____

_____

_____

_____

_____

_____

_____

_____

_____

_____

_____

_____

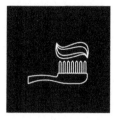

A ROUTINE MOMENT

My husband has always been a person who has not enjoyed last-minute changes. He has always liked a structured, predictable schedule. Regardless of this preference, he has always been able to adapt to spontaneous situations if needed. After all, life is unpredictable, so flexibility is a necessity. Lately, though, I have noticed that he needs a predictable schedule to prevent him from becoming agitated and irritable. His day-to-day routines need to be in place. If we do not follow these routines, one of two things happens: either he becomes angry at me, or he refuses to do anything. What is going on, and what can I do to support him?

Cognitive impairment typically affects a person's short-term and working memory earlier in the disease process than other memory types. A person with impaired short-term and working memory relies on procedural and long-term memory, aka routine memory. Novel events or activities that require the person to adapt and use areas of the brain, such as problem-solving, abstract thinking, or planning, will not be successful. Those areas of the brain will not function well as cognitive impairment progresses.

What activities or events do we focus on if we cannot do novel things? The answer is to operate within a predictable routine because this does not require high amounts of effort from the impaired brain functions. Without a predictable routine, a care partner may notice their loved one exhibits emotions such as avoidance, anger, or withdrawal. In the story above, the husband wants to be successful; however, new situations create a demand that his brain cannot meet. This demand, if unmanageable, causes him to feel out of control and incompetent. A predictable routine removes the demand from the brain's impaired functions, allowing the husband control, independence, and success. A routine can facilitate positive emotions rather than the negative emotions described by the care partner above.

As a care partner, you can support your loved one's success with daily living tasks by allowing these tasks to unfold in the same sequence as your loved one has always completed the job. Another way to support your loved one is to allow the entire day to develop in the same sequence as is typical. One way to determine the usual sequence of your loved one's day or a common task is to journal.

Journaling is a way to determine what sequence worked, what did not, what you and your loved one wish to continue in the future, and what needs to be modified. Writing down steps for a specific task or for actions in the day or week helps replicate these same tasks in the same order in the future. By doing so, we are building procedural memory ("how-to" memory) and allowing the individual with impaired cognition to rely on his or her strength, which is using procedural type of memory for everyday tasks.

Journaling can also serve as an emotional release for any person. It can help us quiet our minds and care for ourselves. By journaling, we increase our awareness of how we are coping with the enormous changes that are taking place in our lives, and this helps us identify any needed support systems not already implemented. Long into the future, these journals can also serve as reminiscing tools and "how-to guides" for outside care partners if the disease progresses to that point.

Routine Moment Takeaways:

- Implement a predictable sequence of events for day-to-day living and each daily task.

- Predictability will allow an individual with cognitive impairment to use his or her intact procedural memory, ensuring success and reducing negative emotions.

- To help attend to the day's simple routines, using a journal or log can help identify the small things that we otherwise may take for granted.

My thoughts:

_____

_____

_____

_____

_____

_____

_____

_____

_____

_____

_____

_____

_____

_____

_____

_____

_____

_____

_____

_____

_____

_____

_____

_____

_____

_____

_____

_____

_____

_____

_____

_____

_____

_____

_____

_____

_____

_____

_____

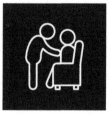

ANTICIPATE THE MOMENT

Betty is living with dementia. She has become angry with her care partners. Each day the care partners come into her apartment to assist her with dressing, but, in Betty's words, "They treat me like a dress-up Barbie and just do it for me." Each day her care partners come in, Betty is already, in her reality, dressed for the day, because she looks at herself and she has clothing on.

Betty says things like "I can do it myself," which the care partners believe is incorrect because if the care partners do not assist her, she does not get dressed and stays in her pajamas all day. The care partners know Betty to be a lady who appreciates her appearance and likes being well dressed. The care partners frequently think they are in a no-win situation. Why do these care partners feel like there is no winning and they are between a rock and a hard place?

Betty, in the story previous, can do things for herself. However, the care partners do not yet understand the tools needed to help her to her best ability. Betty has lost the ability to initiate a task and sequence through all steps. "To the best of someone's ability" means that each person has capabilities, and we assist or support people to use all of the abilities they have. As dementia progresses, these abilities shift. To help someone with dementia to his or her best ability means that you only fill the gaps in cognition that are not firing well, rather than taking over the whole task. With each person, and at each cognitive level, there is a "just right" with the level of cueing and assistance a care partner provides.

In Betty's situation, maybe she needs a caregiver to set up supplies so that there is a visual cue to get the task complete. Perhaps she needs the caregiver to set up and then provide a simple, direct, loving, and respectful cue to start the task. Or maybe she needs the caregiver to break the task of getting dressed into smaller steps and then give a kind, verbal direction with each step. In the later stages of the disease, she may need her care partners to assist her physically yet still cue her so she can feel she is still participating in the task and is not a Barbie doll being bent and twisted without her acceptance. As you can see, a care partner needs to complement and build on loved ones' abilities, rather than overshadowing and taking away these abilities.

Our ability to anticipate and meet the needs of our loved one with dementia is critical, especially since the person's capabilities to plan and initiate are going to be impaired almost immediately. If our loved one's cognitive impairment is progressive, his or her needs will change. The executive functions within an individual's brain, as we learned earlier, are like the stoplights that direct traffic. These are the functions that tell the "workers" what to do and when to do it. When these functions are not correctly working, the individual will look as if she cannot complete a task, as we saw with Betty. However, the reality is that she may just need a little cue or a nudge to do so. This cue takes the traffic controllers' place in her brain so the "workers" can begin their work.

When anticipating the needs of a loved one, first, we need to know the person's preferred routines. Then we can be "the person's brain" and be the substitute for the failing "traffic controllers". As dementia progresses, we may need to substitute for some of the "workers" as well. Filling small pieces or roles, rather than taking over a whole task, can help the individual feel successful each day. This anticipation allows the care partners to "do with" and not "do for," which will enable individuals like Betty to keep their pathways firing, maintain their abilities, their dignity, and their feelings of self-worth. Think about it as complementing, rather than controlling, your loved one's actions.

Varying the type and amount of assistance is called grading. This concept was introduced when we were discussing foundational insights into the brain in a previous section. Grading is the ability to make a situation more or less challenging to suit the person's needs. Think of the road gradient at the side of the road, sloping gently until the road ends. The amount of assistance needs to be gradually graded so as not to take away a person's remaining abilities or cause the individual to "fall off the road." We want it to be a smooth, slow transition, one baby step at a time. Grading a task or engagement is necessary to create success and help a person feel confident, dignified, and preserved in his or her self-worth.

The first step to grading is to identify your loved one's specific needs, either through trial and error or through a functional cognitive assessment from a professional, such as an occupational therapist. For example, an occupational therapist might identify a deficit in planning or initiating a task. These processes are the first cognitive functions that need grading to ensure success. Assisting your loved one by anticipating and meeting his or her preferred needs is one of the critical moments requiring your insight.

If we, as care partners, do not learn how to grade tasks and engagements for our loved ones throughout the day, we risk fostering negative emotions and excess disability. Excess disability refers to our loved ones losing function faster than they otherwise would have, given the disease. Help your loved ones preserve their full range of abilities by complementing their actions while performing day-to-day tasks. As their capabilities shift, anticipate where you may need to provide a cue or assistance and meet that need before they encounter a problem due to impaired cognition.

Frequently, in the early stages of dementia, a person will experience depressive symptoms. Depressive symptoms could result from feeling helpless or hopeless, or lacking self-worth, for example. However, in the early stages of the disease, when the initiation of action and abstract thinking are the central impairments, what if this isolation or lack of participation we see is not depression? What if a person's withdrawal or perceived withdrawal from previously enjoyed and meaningful tasks and engagements are the "traffic controllers" not firing as they should? What if Betty wishes that she could still initiate and let others know what she still wants to do, but she gets overwhelmed by open-ended invites and needs a little nudge in the right direction? What if we can do something to anticipate her dysfunction and complement her previous function and desire to be social?

Too often, we assume that what we see on the outside is reality, and we do not dig deep enough to help our loved one maintain the person he or she was and still is. A person's perceived disinterest may actually be the individual saying, "I'm not sure how to do this any longer, and I don't want to make a fool of myself." We can help bridge this gap by assisting with initiation in a polite, respectful, and loving way, helping to maintain the person we love, who will be *Ever-Present* with our support.

To make these supportive cues successful, the care partner will need to paint a picture with an invitation or cue to help Betty use her concrete brain. Using concrete, descriptive language and throwing in a little love and excitement can go a long way to foster acceptance and a desire to say yes to what you are requesting or suggesting. At times, as you anticipate and meet your loved one's cognitive needs, you may feel pushy or bossy; however, you are not! Keep a focus on the person, your loved one, along with a filter of acceptance, respect, love, and grace. Remember his or her preferred roles, routines, hobbies, and preferences from the past. If these things are in focus, you will never force your loved one to do something he or she does not want to do; you will merely be assisting the person to do as he or she would have before the disease. You are adapting to the disability and complementing the person so he or she can live life to the fullest.

In earlier stages of dementia, an appearance of avoidance or missing tasks signifies that a care partner needs to begin to anticipate and meet a loved one's needs. In later stages of dementia, the signs and symptoms you look for to know how to cue your loved one turn into behaviors, expressions, or gestures that may look odd to you but are communication from your loved one. The person with impaired cognition will begin to communicate in nontraditional ways. For example, if a person needs to use the restroom and has lost the ability to initiate or figure out where the toilet is, she may begin to pace or become frustrated and angry. This pacing is your cue as a care partner that the individual needs you to anticipate her need and help her meet it by complementing the abilities she still maintains. By anticipating her need to use the bathroom, you can use gentle cueing to guide her to the bathroom on a routine basis, thus eliminating these negative behaviors. These negative behaviors were her attempt to communicate a need for more support from you, her care partner, and her loved one.

Anticipate the Moment Takeaways:

- Anticipate your loved ones' needs and the amount and type of support they may need in each situation.

- Plan and provide this assistance in an anticipatory fashion, rather than waiting for the person to have a problem or forget an important task in the day. Provide that "just right" support to avoid negative interactions and emotions. This "just right" support may include:

  » assisting with initiation by setting out supplies as a visual cue,

  » assisting with the initiation or onset of a task through a polite invitation or suggestion,

  » giving polite verbal directions throughout a task or at each new step, or

  » physically helping a loved one with a task while describing your actions throughout (using varying levels of physical assistance).

My thoughts:

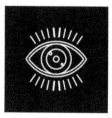

MOLD THE MOMENT

My husband refuses to shave. Even when I tell him to, he gets mad and says he does not need to shave anymore. I have walked him into the bathroom and asked him to do it. I have begged and pleaded, but nothing seems to work. How can I mold this moment and get the desired and necessary outcome of shaving? It is not that I want him to shave. I know he would never have wanted to look scruffy like he is now. I know that if it were not for his dementia, he would be happy to shave. Help!

Planning, to mold a moment to make it desirable, is another insight that a care partner will need to practice and fine-tune. Imagine you are planning a fun night out with a significant other or friends. It is a surprise, and you want everything to be perfect. What do you do? You start planning, down to the very last detail, so that when that person arrives, he or she does not have to think about a thing. The person gets to come and experience the opportunity you have planned and laid out. Planning like this is what we must do as care partners for a person with dementia.

People's ability to process the world around them changes as they develop any type of cognitive dysfunction. A simple task like shaving, using the shower, or a social situation like a previously enjoyed coffee group can become challenging or difficult due to this change in perception. As care partners, we can anticipate this change in people's needs, as we just previously learned, and do more planning to create an experience that will be pleasurable and meaningful for our loved ones. Molding any moment by planning and adding "sensory touches" to improve satisfaction can be helpful in many moments. However, this molding of a moment is especially necessary if you anticipate an upcoming difficult moment.

One example of molding the moment could include setting up a bathroom to be warm and inviting. Play appropriate music and use aromatherapy to create a barber- or spa-type experience. Set up the environment with a person's favorite supplies that smell familiar, towels that are warm and soft, and water that has already run and is warm right from the start. After all this planning and molding of the moment, then invite or cue your loved one to come and experience this barbershop or spa rather than saying, "Come take a shower." Turn each moment into an experience rather than a task or a chore. Create intrigue and motivation; this facilitates participation and acceptance of assistance. Through our invite, the desired thought we are trying to provoke in our loved one is, "That sounds so wonderful. I want to check it out."

Side note: a fascinating fact is that our sense of smell connects with our long-term memory. Smelling the same aftershave that our loved one has used for forty-plus years can trigger memories of shaving or a favorite barbershop, thus assisting with initiating and implementing the activity.

A second example of molding the moment may be at mealtime. Nicely set the table; use a tablecloth of appealing color (but not too distracting). Have your loved one in the kitchen while you prepare so he or she can smell the food cooking and get hungry. Reminisce about food, the person's favorites, and what you are cooking. Use descriptive language so that your loved one can have "food on the brain." The clearer the picture you can paint with your words through descriptive language while reminiscing, the better. Play soft music in the background that is enjoyable, to create a pleasant mood.

Molding a moment has two components.

1. The sensory component, which is helpful to assist in a pleasant perception of the moment. Facilitate the activation of as many senses as you can.

2. The anticipatory component: setting up the environment for success by anticipating (as we just learned prior) what you or your loved one will need in that moment and having those items readily available. The environment plays a crucial role in creating success for the moment. As the care partner, you are the producer mixing the backup singers (yourself) and track (atmosphere) to make the music as a whole the best it can be. Help create beautiful music with your loved one, who is the lead singer.

Mold the Moment Takeaways:

- Consider the sensory components of a task and anticipate the materials needed. Incorporate these sensory components with the necessary materials to create a pleasing sensory experience.

- Use pleasant and familiar smells to trigger positive memories and aid in initiating and executing the desired activity.

- Use an irresistible invitation to an experience rather than a boring suggestion to complete a task to encourage performance.

My thoughts:

_____

_____

_____

_____

_____

_____

_____

_____

_____

_____

_____

_____

_____

_____

_____

_____

_____

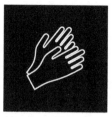

EMBRACE THE MOMENT

I just attended a dementia class. The speaker was great and had fantastic ideas to help me be a better care partner for my wife, Janene. I was excited to come home and try the tricks and ideas I had learned. So, I woke up, I molded the moment, anticipated her needs, and I thought I did everything correctly. But it still did not work. I had a rather difficult moment, and I was disheartened. Why didn't it work?

When we try our best to anticipate and mold moments to make them pleasant, there will still be moments that do not work out as we hope. Since the brain is such a complex organ, we will never be able to anticipate and plan 100 percent successfully. The fantastic abilities in our brain—reasoning, judgment, planning, emotional regulation, problem-solving, sequencing, and processing of the world around us, to name a few—all may begin to experience various degrees of dysfunction. When this happens, it is impossible to completely know what is going on in a brain outside our own. All we as care partners can do is try. As Thomas H. Palmer stated once, "If at first, you don't succeed, try, try, and try again." If you are trying, you are succeeding!

We need to remember that we are watching a situation from the outside, looking in. We will never be able to get into another person's brain so that we can see, feel, and experience the world precisely from the other individual's point of view. In some moments, our thoughts might be "this is terrible," or "this needs to stop," or we might be embarrassed by what is happening. It is only natural for us to stop an uncomfortable situation, fix a disaster, or hide a mistake. However, because we have such deep love for our family members with dementia, we must embrace the moment at times. We need to reassess and think, "Is this a big deal?"; "Is this causing harm to anyone or anything?"; "So what?" If no one is in danger, and property is not vulnerable to destruction, it may be best to let the situation unfold as it will. As with most life problems, you sometimes must pick your battles, embrace the moment, and move on.

By taking a step back, embracing the moment, and carefully observing, we can learn something critical about our loved ones and how they experience the world. By not trying to change each moment to suit what we would hold as our ideal, we understand how to facilitate successful moments in the future, days, months, or years. The learning we go through as we embrace the moment is SUCCESS!

Embrace the Moment Takeaways:

- Sometimes we must decide if the moment is a big deal that needs intervention or if the moment can carry on outside of our ideological perception.
- If a misused word harms no one during a conversation or the counter-top is being washed for the hundredth time that day, we may need to accept this for what it is, learn about our loved one, and move on.

My thoughts:

_____

_____

_____

_____

_____

_____

_____

_____

_____

_____

_____

_____

_____

_____

_____

_____

_____

_____

_____

_____

_____

_____

_____

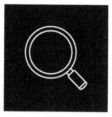

STUDY THE MOMENT

Shortly after breakfast each day, my wife Violet begins to take off her shirt. It is the middle of winter, and our house can be rather chilly. I do not want her to get cold, so I tell her to put it back on. Plus, she needs to wear a shirt, for heaven's sake! But when I ask her to put her shirt back on, she becomes angry with me and often yells while continuing to take the garment off. Sometimes other clothes are removed as well. Why does she do this, and what can I do to make sure she stays warm and dressed appropriately?

Because we cannot climb into our loved ones' brains to see and understand their perspectives firsthand, we need to be observant. We must become detectives. Our loved ones will communicate, behave, and present themselves differently than we have ever witnessed. The outward appearance of what we think we are seeing may not reflect a loved one's real intent. We must patiently study, analyze, and problem-solve through situations with our loved ones' perspectives in mind. Enhance your attention to detail and your critical-thinking skills. Remain supportive and patient as you investigate through active listening and observation.

Difficult moments and also not-so-tricky moments can serve as educational tools for a caregiver if patient observation and investigation are applied. Become a student in learning your loved one's new experience of the world. Be a detective and dig deep, past what appears on the surface. Often there is a root cause that explains the situation in a much different way than what we thought we saw with our own eyes.

Dealing with these more difficult moments can feel overwhelming, and thinking about slowing down so we can study them (when we are in the middle of the moment) can be extremely challenging. The more challenging the moment is, the more tempting it will be to step in and react promptly. Rather than quickly *reacting*, it is beneficial to *study and respond*.

Consider keeping a journal. As we discussed earlier, journaling can be a helpful way to study and respond. This journal about day-to-day moments, routines, and preferences can help us survey and reflect at the end of the day when our minds are clear, and we can concentrate. Unpacking a difficult moment at the end of the day will help us not feel overwhelmed when a similar situation arises. Give yourself and your loved one the grace needed to get through the difficult moments. Reflect after the fact to see if you can identify a root cause. The grace you extend will help you remain focused on the *Ever-Present* person you love despite the disability of dementia.

When in these difficult moments, you will notice expressive communication from your loved one, sometimes referred to as "behaviors." A behavior is merely everything we do. It is how a person acts or conducts him or herself, how he or she performs or responds to a situation or a stimulus. Many dementia care courses teach that behavior is communication. A quote from Paul Watzlowick states this perfectly, "You cannot, not communicate. Every behavior is a form of communication. Because behavior does not have a counterpart (there is no anti-behavior), it is not possible to not communicate." Keeping this quote in your mind as a care partner of someone with cognitive impairment is vitally important, especially in these difficult moments.

A behavioral expression is our loved one's way of communicating to us in a nontraditional way. As we learned in the foundational communication insight previously, this nontraditional way of communicating will become our loved one's primary form of communication. It is always meaningful and has a purpose; we need to slow down enough to observe, hear, listen, and understand what people are trying to tell us through their behavior.

Think of the expressive communication from your loved one as if you are learning a new language. It takes years to master a second language. You learn bits and pieces, try to apply them, say things wrong at times, misinterpret things, modify what you know, and then continue. Learning our loved one's "new language" is no different. The communication center of the person's brain is impaired by this disease process, thus requiring our loved one to use a new language. We must learn to speak people's language to effectively communicate and help them navigate their unique experience of the world. However, as with learning any new language, this will take trial and error, practice, and patience. Accepting and providing grace through this process is a great start to help you learn this new language effectively, without getting frustrated and overwhelmed. Accept the fact that you will mess up and need to adjust. Accept that your loved one will mess up, to which you will also need to adjust. Provide yourself and your loved one grace in these moments so that you can maintain the composure that is required each day.

If we refuse to learn the new language of our loved ones and try to stop every moment that is not ideal, we are effectively "clipping their vocal cords." Since this is our loved ones' way of communicating, by stifling all the moments (that to us may seem odd or difficult), we are taking away their ability to communicate. Fight this urge and instead study the moment so you can get to a root cause.

To help you navigate through this new study of your loved one, here is a list of different needs and questions you can ask yourself as you are studying this new language. Keep in mind, asking "why" after you think you may have found a root cause might uncover something even more profound. After you believe you have identified a solution by asking "why," ask it again!

Is your loved one communicating a basic or physical need?

1. Does the person need to use the bathroom?
2. Has the person had adequate output lately of both bowel and bladder?
3. Is he or she hungry or thirsty?
4. Is your loved one uncomfortable? Stiff from sitting too long or being stagnant? Achy from walking or moving too much?
5. Is the person in pain?
6. Is the person too hot or too cold?

7. Does your loved one have all his or her sensory devices to maximize sensory systems (i.e., hearing aids, glasses, dentures, etc.)?

Is your loved one communicating a psychological need? As discussed earlier, people have six basic psychological needs—love, attachment, comfort, identity, occupation, and inclusion. These need to be at the forefront of our brains as we study the moment.

1. Is the person bored?

2. Is your loved one lonely?

3. Is the person scared or fearful?

4. Is your loved one seeking comfort, familiarity, or security?

5. Is he or she seeking human interaction or touch?

Is your loved one communicating an environmental need?

1. Is the environment too loud or too quiet?

2. Is the environment too dark or too bright?

3. Are there shadows in the environment that are creating a misperception?

4. Are there sounds in the environment that may be unexpected or startling?

5. Is the typical routine or environment out of place?

6. Is there a proper balance of stimuli in the environment? Meaning, is there a rotation of stimulating moments and calming moments to allow your loved one to refuel his or her mental energy after depletion?

Is your loved one communicating a need from you or another care partner that is required to help the person succeed?

1. Is the care partner moving at a reasonable speed, not too fast or too slow for the individual's processing speed?

2. Is the care partner "doing with" rather than "doing for" the individual; exhibiting a partnership of care, rather than taking over care, to maintain autonomy?

3. Is the care partner building trust and empathy with each interaction, even if the individuals know each other well?

4. Is the care partner aware of and speaking positively with his or her body language, facial expressions, and nonverbals so the individual can receive them in the best way?

5. Is the care partner following the individual's preferred routine?

The lists above may be overwhelming. However, this is not the intent. The intent is to demonstrate the complexity of what your loved one may be communicating. The lists emphasize the importance of trial and error. You will have clear moments in which you will know what your loved one needs. In contrast, you will have some puzzling moments where you will need to work through problems with your loved one, trialing different solutions until you come up with the right one.

In the example at the beginning of this section, the husband described his wife disrobing shortly after breakfast each day. Let us hear from him about his conclusion after studying and reflecting on this difficult moment.

As I studied Violet's tendency to disrobe after breakfast and reflected on this consistent moment we were experiencing, I remembered that she always used the bathroom after breakfast. I did not notice this before because she would simply walk herself to the bathroom. However, due to her dementia, she must not be able to get herself there independently any longer and is unable to tell me she still has that need. Her new language may be trying to verbalize that she still has this need. She is uncomfortable and unsure how to fix her discomfort. I decided to escort her to the bathroom roughly 10 minutes after breakfast each day, before she began disrobing. It worked! She stopped undressing after breakfast and our difficult moment subsided.

To help you understand the complexity of "why" and the need to dig deep, the same scenario described above may have a completely different meaning to another person. As a therapist, I have worked with many individuals who exhibit disrobing. One in particular that comes to mind was disrobing because her skin was dry and itchy. She was also cold. She knew that her skin was uncomfortable (dry, itchy, cold) but didn't know how to fix it. Thus her communication method was taking off clothing. As individuals with intact cognition, we may see this as counterproductive and unexplainable. However, to this lady, it was 100 percent productive and perfectly understandable.

Through trial and error, we identified that if we were diligent at applying lotion to the woman's skin morning and night, as well as dressing her in a turtleneck and overshirt to help keep her warm, her disrobing ceased. As care partners, we needed to take another look at history, routines, and preferences and attempt to meet any unmet needs.

As you can see, a situation that looks one way to us (the outsiders) may have two very different meanings to the person who communicates the need. Always remember, if you are trying, you are succeeding.

Study the Moment Takeaways:

- A situation may not always be as it appears on the surface. There is typically an underlying reason for challenging behavior.
- Be a detective. Keep a journal, note patterns, remember old routines, and slowly peel back the layers of the moment so you can uncover the underlying need. By meeting that underlying need, you may be able to avoid some challenging moments.

Additional Learning:
See Appendix A for more specific examples of behavioral expressions and identified reasons for these challenging behaviors.

My thoughts:

_____

_____

_____

_____

_____

_____

_____

_____

_____

_____

_____

_____

_____

_____

_____

_____

_____

_____

_____

_____

_____

_____

_____

_____

_____

_____

_____

_____

_____

_____

_____

_____

_____

_____

_____

_____

_____

_____

_____

_____

_____

_____

_____

_____

_____

_____

_____

_____

_____

_____

_____

_____

_____

_____

_____

_____

_____

_____

_____

_____

_____

_____

_____

_____

_____

SAVE THE MOMENT

A new pastor greeted Lillian. Lillian believed this pastor was her pastor from years ago in her hometown. This new pastor came to say hello and to meet her for the first time. He wanted to see how she was settling into her new apartment in a senior living community and to welcome her to the community. Lillian had just moved to this apartment from a neighboring town. Her pastor from her hometown was of similar build and appearance as this new pastor greeting her. She thought she knew him. Due to her cognitive impairment, she did not recognize that the new pastor was not the previous pastor who had helped her cope with her son's death about two years earlier.

Lillian's daughter came to visit a while later and said, "Well, Mom, it was so nice of your new pastor to come and visit." To which Lillian replied, "New pastor? He is not new. I've known him for years. He helped me through your brother's passing. When he left, he even gave me a hug because he remembered me so well."

Lillian's daughter saw that she was becoming upset and confused, embarrassed and offended by this new pastor hugging her since they had only just met. Lillian's daughter tried to "save face" for Lillian as she explained that it was a new pastor, yes, but he was a nice man, so it was okay that they hugged. (Lillian was typically a person that reserved hugs for family and people she knew very well.)

There was now a misunderstanding. Lillian pondered this new versus old pastor in her life. Because of the embarrassment she felt, she would snap at everyone who would approach her. Staff in her new living community would assist her, and she would be startled easily. Seeing her unease, the staff would attempt to explain and try to calm her. Each attempt to use reasoning and logic to explain to Lillian what had happened made things worse and not better. All the "explaining" by staff and her daughter (done out of concern for Lillian) was not proving helpful.

As you can see from this example, explaining something with logic and reasoning in "our reality" can prove to be of little help and may even make difficult situations worse. The best-case scenario is that our logical explanation of reality does sink in. The countereffect of this is that the person living with impairment then feels embarrassed or foolish because he or she forgot, misunderstood, or made a mistake. This only emphasizes that the person's brain is not functioning correctly and contributes to feelings of frustration, worthlessness, or loss of self.

Our goal is to build our loved one up, not break someone like Lillian down. Her brain is already telling her she is missing things or not thinking correctly. She doesn't need an outsider to point it out. Often isolation or refusal to partake in previously enjoyed social engagements is a product of these feelings. So, what do we do if reality orientation only creates negative feelings that turn into a downward spiral?

In these situations, as tricky as they may be, we need to "save the moment," as Lillian's granddaughter will do when we finish her story below. Rather than placing the blame on Lillian's poor memory, her granddaughter figures out a way to enter Lillian's reality and fix the mistake by placing the blame back onto herself. A superhero moment such as this is where we, as care partners, get to swoop in and "save the day." We get the opportunity to use our imagination and put new puzzle pieces into place to save face for our loved ones. We can do this by placing any embarrassment or blame onto ourselves, even when we know we are not to blame. Here is the rest of the story, when Lillian's granddaughter saved the moment by blaming herself and removing Lillian's uneasiness.

Lillian's granddaughter was told by her mother (Lillian's daughter) what had happened and the aftermath of this simple misunderstanding. Lillian's daughter said that it was difficult to redirect Lillian no matter what anyone did or said.

Lillian's granddaughter wanted to help. She called Lillian and said, "Grandma, I screwed up! The other day a pastor came to visit you. I had asked your pastor to come to visit to see how you were doing. He had called me and said he could not make it, so I had another pastor fill in for him. But I forgot to call you to tell you a different pastor was coming. He almost looks like a twin of your old pastor. I messed up, and I should have called you to tell you a different pastor was coming. One hundred percent my fault." Her grandmother replied, "Oh, lil' sweetheart, it's okay. It was not a big deal. I appreciated his visit; he was a nice man."

After the "save the day" moment described above, Lillian stopped snapping and getting angry at little things. Her psychological and emotional needs were met and understood by her granddaughter. She saved the day for Lillian by taking the blame and embarrassment off of Lillian's shoulders, improving Lillian's perception and salvaging her feelings of dignity and self-worth.

Life is complicated. Living with cognitive impairment adds further complication, and an ability to "save the moment" can help minimize some of the complexity you may experience in more difficult moments. Throughout this complicated life we live, we interact daily with people. This interaction sometimes goes as we expect. In other exchanges, we walk away thinking, "Well, that didn't go the way I thought." These perplexing moments become more frequent when we interact with a person who lives with dementia.

There is one rule of thumb we need to consider. When reasoning and logic become impaired by cognitive decline, a person's reality shifts; the individual experiences the world differently, as we learned. The rule of thumb is that a person's perception of reality is true to him or her, regardless of how illogical or untrue it appears to an outsider. There is nothing we as an external factor can do to shift or change the individual's reality back to our standard. Thus, when interacting, we need to remember to read and respond with love and patience, rather than react with emotion, even in emotionally charged situations. By reading and responding, we consciously make an effort to promote or preserve a loved one's dignity and build his or her self-worth. This ability to slow down and respond rather than react is a way to "save the day" if we are in a challenging position with a loved one.

Often these more emotionally charged or challenging situations arise out of a misperception. Difficulty with memory, emotional processing or regulation, abstract thinking, and visual perception (just to name a few) contribute to a possible misperception. Something in the external world (a person or the environment) or something within themselves (a basic need, an emotional need, or a psychological need) has created a misperception of the current situation in the person's reality. A straightforward example of this may be an individual who watches a heartbreaking news story, like a car accident, and then develops anxious feeling each time the person sees a car driving outside. Another example may be an individual who hears children screaming while playing but does not actually see the incident happening, so the person begins talking about how children are crying or being harmed.

As we discussed in "mold the moment," we can use ourselves, others around us, and the environment to shape a moment in both positive and negative ways. This molding can help an individual feel validated in his or her feelings, emotions, and perceptions, and this is the key to "saving the day." If a person like Lillian is upset, empathize with that feeling. If she is excitable/anxious, react as though you understand the anxiousness and validate it. If she is sad, grieve with her. Allow your loved one to feel the emotion she is feeling by feeling it yourself. Then you are truly present in that place with her. It is of utmost importance that you hear, listen, and understand what you are receiving from her verbal and nonverbal communication.

To demonstrate another example of saving the moment, read on.

A person was living in a community specifically designed for those with cognitive impairment. This person was female, and she did not like "these strangers watching me shower." A few staff members decided to try a new approach to encourage her to shower. They needed the person to know that they were present to help and that it was okay to allow the help. They needed to build her trust.

One staff member went in to begin the woman showering. When the person became upset at this staff member, a second staff member came in and said, "Oh goodness, is she bothering you? Let me kick her out; you don't need to be bothered. I can help you with this since I know how to respect your privacy. I have helped you before." This staff member then escorted the other staff member out.

The second staff member became the "good cop" in the situation, and the first staff member was the "bad cop" (for lack of better words). The individual with impairment in this situation experienced a fight-or-flight reaction due to feeling threatened or uncomfortable. By swooping in and "saving the day" through the good cop interaction, the second staff member validated the woman's feelings so she could then trust the person to help her shower.

Validation of the emotions expressed in any given moment is the absolute key to navigating these challenging moments. Even if it is a misperception on behalf of the person with the impairment, it is that person's reality to which we must adjust. All human beings need to feel validated in what they are thinking and feeling; this is especially true for those who have limited reasoning and logic. People with impaired cognition are unable to talk themselves through these emotional situations. We partner with them if we keep ourselves calm and rational, joining them in their reality. We can then respond rather than react and validate the individual to get through the moment.

Save the Moment Takeaways:

- The person living with cognitive impairment cannot come back to our reality.
- As humans with intact cognition, we have the mental ability to shift our perspective and enter our loved one's reality, regardless of how illogical it may seem.
- By joining our loved one's reality, validating the experienced emotions, and solving the perceived problem, we gain trust and agreement from our loved one.

My thoughts:

_____

_____

_____

_____

_____

_____

_____

_____

_____

_____

_____

_____

_____

My thoughts:

SHIFT THE MOMENT

Let me introduce you to someone who previously managed a restaurant and enjoyed reading the newspaper, Kenny. If there was a newspaper around, Kenny wanted to catch up on his hometown's latest happenings. He also liked checking on all his patrons in his "restaurant." These patrons were not actual restaurant patrons but were individuals trying to eat their meals in the living community they shared with Kenny. These individuals did not appreciate his check-ins.

The care partners felt conflicted. Should they allow Kenny to be in his reality and "check his patrons" (because, after all, he wasn't hurting anyone)? Was the risk of making him angry too great to intervene? However, "his patrons" did not like his checks, and an altercation between Kenny and a fellow resident was a real possibility without intervention.

The solution: when care partners would see Kenny finishing up with his meal before he stood up from the table, they would go over, clear his plate, and exchange it for a newspaper. This newspaper served to grab his attention, and it was something that was motivating to him. Handing him the paper was enough to distract him, and reading the newspaper was then the full redirection he needed to be distracted from his perceived patrons. This redirection also gave everyone else time to finish their meals.

Distraction is the first essential skill we will discuss to "shift the moment." Distraction is the ability to shift a person's brain quickly from one topic to another. The art of distraction is necessary when a person may be stuck on a topic or action that is possibly intrusive to others, or themselves, at the moment, and it needs to cease quickly to prevent it from worsening. The key a care partner needs to keep in mind is that this distraction will result in the individual reverting right back, if not followed up by some type of full redirection away from the previous topic or action.

Redirection is the second essential skill we need to remember to "shift the moment." Redirection is shifting a person's brain entirely away from the previous topic to a new topic for a more extended time. Distraction is quick, a simple attention-grabber. Redirection complements distraction by maintaining attention until the person's focus shifts to a new topic.

To distract a person from a topic or action, we need to consider two things to get a person to "want" to do anything: attention and motivation. Thus, to shift gears quickly, we need to think through attention and motivation for the person we are attempting to help. (Fun fact about memory: attention and motivation are also two important factors to facilitate memory, along with emotion.)

Moments of high emotional intensity are more challenging to overcome with distraction. Due to this, we must add two more pieces to the puzzle before distracting the individual if we want the distraction and following redirection to be successful. We must validate the person's feelings and then deflect from whatever created the negative emotion.

As we discussed in previous moments, validating our loved one's feelings will be critical once again! Strong validation, followed by appropriate distraction, will be more successful than merely attempting to distract in these moments of high emotional intensity. If you try to distract without first validating any negative emotions, it will send the wrong signal to your loved one. The person will feel that you "are not understanding" or are trying to "brush his or her feelings aside." If your loved one feels this way, a strong adverse emotional reaction may present itself, and the situation will quickly escalate. A vicious cycle ensues with each of our heightened emotions. We find ourselves in a reactionary phase rather than a study and respond phase. It is up to us to pause, calm, think, and respond rather than react.

Here is an example to consider when thinking about these two add-ons to distraction in highly emotional situations: validation and deflection.

Bob comes out of his room after getting dressed. His shirt is buttoned in the wrong order, and he is frustrated! He knows something is wrong. You have two choices. You could react and say, "Bob, you buttoned your shirt wrong; let me help." This reaction would then trigger Bob to feel embarrassed. You did not validate his evident frustration. You added to it by saying he did something wrong.

Or you could use the techniques discussed, and you could walk up and say, "Oh my goodness, Bob, you look frustrated. These shirts!! I always struggle with this brand too. Let me see if I can use the tricks that I've learned to help you out." Having this dialogue will allow him to feel validated, and Bob will feel he is not alone in his struggles.

In this instance, if you selected option two for your response, you validated Bob's feeling of frustration to distract him to a more positive emotional place. You deflected what he may have perceived as blame on himself onto an object in the environment. You successfully preserved his dignity by deflecting away from his disability and redirecting to something both he and you could be frustrated about together! At this moment, you helped him feel like he was not the problem and shifted the problem to something exterior, the shirt. You gained his trust by sharing his feelings of frustration.

As we shift a moment and deflect from disabilities, we need to be cautious that we do not take away abilities an individual still has remaining. There will be moments when the care partner will be worried or concerned that a loved one may encounter a problem. In these moments, it is tempting to step in before the individual needs assistance. As we discussed in *Anticipate the Moment*, we must anticipate a problem and meet a need before it arises. However, this is when we know for sure the person's abilities are failing based on previous moments. If we step in too early, we potentially stop pathways in the brain from functioning due to the care partner "doing for them" rather than "doing with them."

This caution will be a continuous process that the care partner will need to keep in the back of his or her mind. It will be a trial-and-error process: allowing as much independence as possible, only stepping in after a problem arises or when we know we have had a problem in the past, but stepping in before an emotional outburst. Finding that "just right moment to intervene" will be homework for you as a care partner. Be patient and give yourself grace as you navigate this "just right"; it is not an easy task, but this homework will pay off tenfold once mastered.

Shift the Moment Takeaways:

- Using distraction can help quickly stop or divert your loved one away from a place, person, task, or object. Remember, if you want this distraction to be useful, it must coincide with full redirection.

- Using an appropriate, motivating, and timely distraction can prevent a domino effect of negative behaviors and emotions from arising.

- The addition of validation (sharing your loved one's feelings with him or her) and deflection (shifting blame away from your loved one's mistake) serve as two additions in your ever-growing tool belt to improve the effect of distraction.

My thoughts:

_____

_____

_____

_____

_____

CONFIRM THE MOMENT

I care for my sister with dementia, Clara. Her husband passed away five years ago, but she does not remember that this event occurred. She often says, "I need to find Bill." I always tell her that Bill died five years ago to help her understand reality, but she becomes so upset that I cannot comfort her. We have this same interaction nearly every day, sometimes multiple times a day. How can I reason with her to help her understand that Bill is not here anymore?

Sometimes the best thing to do is a mixture of embracing, studying, saving, and shifting: confirm the moment or the feelings in the moment rather than refuting them. Even though this is best, it may sound like a more complicated way to move through moments in the day; however, don't give up. Keep reading to add a greater explanation to this key in the moment.

Saying "no" is often the comment that flows the easiest from our mouths. A naturally flowing "no, but…" comes from a logical place in our minds of right/wrong, good/bad, yes/no, or things are either one way, not another. If you have raised or cared for children in your lifetime, saying "no" feels like it is almost second nature to a care partner because we want children to grow into good people. However, if you find yourself saying "no" in this current stage of life while assisting a loved one with dementia, you will find it to be ineffective.

As we learned in *Study the Moment,* there is always a purpose and reason for what our loved one is showing us. If we accept that there is a purpose and reason for each interaction, saying "no" refutes our loved one's thoughts or feelings.

Saying "no" tells the person his or her communicative intent is pointless. We need to remember there will be realities to the person with dementia that we cannot see or understand. These realities will appear odd and illogical to us, and we may say "no" to reason and explain the facts that we know. In our attempts to clarify reality, we need to remember that the person's truth is different from ours, and refuting his or her truth is not helpful.

Negative words like "no" are common, notably so when dementia has significantly shifted the way our loved one experiences his or her world, as in Clara's world in the example above. (These negative words include any time we negate one of our loved one's thoughts; it does not necessarily have to be the actual word "no.") Negative words create defensiveness in a person that will lead to difficult moments. Keep in mind that the tone and inflection of a person's voice change when a negative word like "no" is said or when we refute our loved one's thoughts. That intonation change contributes to the moment becoming difficult.

An alternative to "no…but" is a "yes…and." Finding a yes is key to confirm the moment and help the person with dementia feel validated in his or her thoughts and feelings. Find something you can agree on and then, if needed, redirect to something else. We need to stop creating barriers, shutting down our loved ones' thoughts and actions. Instead, we must support our loved ones by confirming their thoughts and actions. This way, we can continue to build on what they have begun and help them get through the moment feeling successful and accomplished rather than belittled and incorrect.

> *To continue with Clara's story, when Clara says, "I need to find Bill," Clara's sister could say, "Oh, I love Bill. What do you remember most about Bill? When you two first met, he drove up to our house in his old blue car. Let's go find some pictures of that old blue car." Or, "I miss Bill when he is gone too. Tell me about when you and Bill first met. Did you like him right from the start? Was it love at first sight?"*

Another example of turning a traditional "no" moment to a "yes" moment (with the intent of confirming rather than refuting our loved one's thoughts, feelings, or actions) might be as follows. Let's pretend that we know an individual has already eaten lunch; however, she continues to come up to you and say, "I would like some lunch." Rather than saying, "No, you already had lunch," you could say, "Yes, you must feel hungry. I get hungry a lot too; let's see what we can find to eat." And then, if you know the person has already eaten lunch, you can find something small for her to snack on.

One last example would be a loved one who comes to you and is angry at another person for "doing something" that you are sure never happened. You want to reason with the person to help him or her not be offended. After all, being offended does not create pleasant feelings. Why would we confirm a negative or unpleasant feeling? Wouldn't it be easier to help this person feel not offended? A brain that can reason could understand this explanation. However, in a cognitively impaired brain that is unable to reason and thus is driven by feelings alone, we need to confirm or validate these feelings to help shift them in a more pleasant direction.

Refuting an emotion or feeling is like pouring gasoline on a fire. In a situation where someone is feeling wronged, rather than saying, "No, they didn't do that; they would never hurt you," you could say, "Yes, I sometimes feel angry and afraid too." Following this validating "yes" with redirection and a simple explanation will shape the person's feelings positively. In short, these interactions need to start with a "yes," not a "no."

In the above examples, our reality would have told us that a "no" with an explanation would be the most logical thing to say. However, if our loved one's brain is not responding well to logic because her brain is experiencing the world differently, we need to use a validating "yes." We agree with the feeling because feelings are genuine and drive behavior!

Continue the Moment Takeaways:

- Challenge your thought process when you automatically think "no" or want to refute an answer.

- Find creative ways to say "yes," in a manner of speaking.

- When you have difficulty confirming the situation, you still need to confirm your loved one's feelings. Using a yes response, such as agreeing with a certain feeling or situation, your loved one feels validated. Using other techniques discussed throughout this book will then be more effective.

My thoughts:

_____

_____

_____

_____

_____

_____

_____

_____

_____

_____

_____

_____

_____

_____

_____

_____

_____

_____

_____

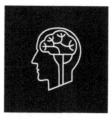

REMEMBER THE MOMENT

My dad, John, has had dementia for years. It has now progressed to a level where I find it challenging to visit with him. I struggle to find conversation because he does not contribute. I find myself having a one-sided conversation during each visit. I often wonder where my dad went, and it makes my heart so sad. Before dementia, he was always so bright and alive, and now he is distant. He has had many memorable experiences in his life, and we have unlimited photo albums that remind me of the life he lived. Sometimes these photo albums bring up an emotional time because life is so different now as he lives with dementia. What do I do? How do I still make our time together meaningful? He is visibly sitting with me when we are together; however, I do not see my dad any longer. Am I correct in thinking that it does not matter as much if I even come to visit daily like I always have?

Living with dementia or living with a loved one with dementia is sometimes described as watching yourself or your loved one disappear, even though both you and the person are still physically present. This description is not incorrect; however, we can choose to see the reality of dementia through a different lens. Rather than seeing an elderly woman who looks like your mother playing with baby dolls, you can choose to see a moment in time where you get to watch the loving, caring, and nurturing way she once took care of you as a child.

Dementia will never be something we can jump up and down about, nor is any other dysfunction that our human bodies experience as they age or encounter the disease. But it also does not have to be a death sentence that we wait to die from moment by moment as the years progress. We can choose to see it for what it is, "a shift in the way we experience the world" (Power, 2010), and rather than feeling bad and waiting to die, we can choose to make the most of the time we have and live. An individual can live through all stages of dementia, and care partners can maximize the function a person has remaining at all stages if they hold tight to the belief that individuals are still present and have abilities, even to the very end.

We can maximize the time we have with our loved one who lives with dementia by becoming fluent in the art of reminiscing. This is a skill that creates meaningful moments and immense joy for both you and your loved one. A simple way to think about reminiscing is to think about recreating past moments of joy using sensory input. To do this, we activate multiple senses while using descriptive storytelling to relive meaningful, joyful moments from the past. Incorporating as many senses as possible triggers more positive memories than verbal conversation or storytelling alone.

To help determine which senses you might incorporate into conversation or storytelling, here are a few examples a care partner might use, using a reminiscence experience about a wedding:

1. Sight—think about what your loved one saw during the experience and use those visual supports during reminiscing. Example: a wedding photo album.
2. Hearing—think about the sounds of the engagement or activity and replicate those if possible. Example: playing the song first danced to at the person's wedding.
3. Taste—think about anything that your loved one could taste in the experience and replicate these sensations if possible. Example: a piece of cake that is similar to the person's wedding cake.
4. Touch—think about the textures that were felt during the experience and replicate those if possible. Example: handling a piece of lace or satin, like a wedding dress or silk tie.
5. Smell—think about the smells that were encountered during the experience and replicate those if possible. Example: smelling old perfume or cologne or a very similar scent.

It is common to attempt to reminisce only through conversation. Conversation, however, requires a two-way street. Furthermore, conversation without anything concrete (something tangible) is exceedingly difficult for a person with dementia. When an individual has difficulty continuing a reciprocal exchange, meaning the "I talk, then you talk," back and forth we typically expect, we tend to stop conversations rather than adapt. The thought of "I don't know why I try to talk; they never talk back" begins to creep in, and there is a strong temptation to give up.

We are quitting too soon if we allow these thoughts to take hold. There are ways to modify the conversation by adding sensory pieces, which will create an experience and may even improve conversational flow. In later stages of dementia, it is possible to progress into a storytelling format of speaking, an almost one-sided type of communication, paired again with sensory pieces to create meaningful memories.

This may sound confusing, but try not to overthink these moments. Close your eyes and remember what you feel, taste, hear, see, or smell. Then think about what items, ingredients, keepsakes, supplies, or elements you could bring to your loved one to recreate these senses. The goal is to create an experience that will facilitate feelings of joy, comfort, excitement, calm, happiness, or love. These positive emotions will be felt by your loved one, even if the person's contribution or visible response is minimal.

Let us return to the daughter above, who was struggling with interaction with her father.

One day Mark's daughter decided to try something to create an experience for her father. She was not ready to let go of meaningful interaction. She looked through their family photo albums and had many fond memories of the snowboarding trips they used to take every year. She brought in the photo album, along with her father's snowboard, helmet, and goggles. She brought in a fan and shaved ice.

She began the experience by playing her father's favorite music that accompanied their car trips. During this, she showed him pictures of the scenery they would view while driving and told him her favorite memories and stories of their travels. She continued by placing the snowboard, helmet, and goggles, one at a time, in her father's lap and hands, assisting him in feeling each one as she told more stories about these trips.

As she told her stories, she turned on the fan while describing the crisp breeze and handed her father the shaved ice while reminiscing about boarding down the mountain and feeling the cold chill of the snow. She successfully recreated their family snowboarding trips for her father. He smiled and even shed a tear of joy as he listened and experienced this meaningful memory with his daughter.

We cannot remove the disease that is creating the impairment. Still, we can choose to shift our thinking from negative to positive and create lasting joy and experiential interaction for ourselves and our loved ones. Remembering and recreating the past moments through reminiscence is an excellent way to help both yourself as the care partner and your loved one LIVE a meaningful life, despite living it in a new way with this disease. Human souls respond to interaction based on the response we receive from another individual. A positive reaction fuels the desire for further contact. The lack of response we feel we receive is why it begins to feel unnatural or difficult to interact with someone living with dementia. The shift that dementia creates impacts how an individual can respond to interaction. The person's responses will become less and less visible.

Nevertheless, the reactions are still present. Never forget, as small as a response may be (blinking, a slight head nod, grunting, a tear, a smirk, smile, or even decreased muscle tension), it is still present. Your loved one is *Ever-Present*. You can be *Ever-Present* in the ever-changing environment that dementia creates.

Remember the Moment Takeaways:

- The power of positive reminiscing cannot be more greatly emphasized in the early, middle, late, and end stages of dementia.
- By engaging our loved one's five senses concerning a positive memory, we can help the person relive fantastic memories. We can use senses to create experiences and interactions that dignify our loved one's *Ever-Present* nature. Joy, happiness, and love are sure to follow.

My thoughts:

_____

_____

_____

_____

_____

_____

_____

_____

_____

_____

_____

_____

_____

_____

_____

_____

_____

_____

_____

REFERENCES

Alzheimer's Association. (March 2020) *2020 Alzheimer's Disease Fact and Figures*. Alzheimer's & Dementia The Journal of the Alzheimer's Association. Volume 16, Issue 3, pgs 391-460. Retrieved from Alzheimer's Association Report. https://alz-journals.onlinelibrary.wiley.com/doi/full/10.1002/alz.12068

Goleman, D. (1998) *Working with Emotional Intelligence*. Bantam Books. Retrieved from The Complete Summary: Working with Emotional Intelligence, by Daniel Goleman. (2010) Soundview Executive Book Summaries (www.summary.com)

Faronbi, S. & Pryor Learning Solutions, Inc. (2018, June 8). Section: Defining Emotional Intelligence & Self-Awareness (pg. 3-8). *Developing Emotional Intelligence* 2018 Conference, Aberdeen, SD, United States.

Kitwood, T. (1997) *Dementia Reconsidered, the Person Comes First*. Open University Press.

Mehrabian, A. (2007). *Nonverbal Communication*. New Brunswick, NJ: Aldine Transaction. Retrieved from Verbal_vs_Non_Verbal_Communication.pdf (workplacestrategiesformentalhealth.com)

Power, G. A. (2010) *Dementia Beyond Drugs: Changing the Culture of Care*. Health Professions Press, Inc.

Warchol, K. & Dementia Care Specialists, Inc. (2016, Jan. 19 & 20) *Dementia Capable Care: Two-Day Foundation & Dementia Care Partner Applications Course* 2016 conference, Bloomington, MN, United States.

Warchol, K. & Dementia Care Specialists, Inc. (2013, April 26 & 27) *Dementia Capable Care: Dementia Therapy Intermediate Course*. 2013 conference, Oak Brook, IL, United States.

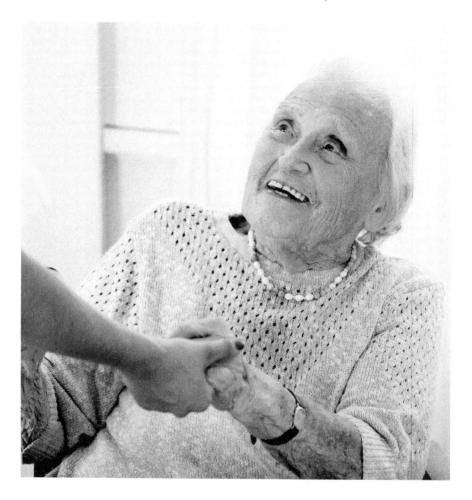

Appendix A:

BEHAVIORAL EXPRESSIONS

Vocal Expression
Aggression
Inappropriate Sexual Expressions
Physical Expressions
Psychological Expressions
Mealtime Expressions

Individuals living with dementia may at times demonstrate "behavioral expressions." These are moments when we as care providers have difficulty understanding these behaviors because they appear to be rather negative or difficult from our viewpoint. As was discussed in *Study the Moment*, we need to learn that these behaviors are our loved ones' attempts at communicating, coping with their impairment, problem-solving, interacting with their world, or feeling overwhelmed or fearful. These behaviors that we have such a difficult time understanding or accepting have a critical purpose!

The key is to shift our view to see the world through our loved ones' eyes, exit our reality, and enter their reality. There is a reason for the behavior you are seeing. Avoid the urge to react and instead respond after studying the entire situation; your loved one, the internal factors, the environment, and external factors. This guide can help you navigate through our observations and study your loved one's new language (behavioral language) to help you see and understand the specific expressional behavior you are witnessing. Understanding the "why" often leads us to know the "what," which assists us in our response.

Each section of the appendix contains these elements:

1. **What type of expression you are seeing**

    a. Divided into categories; examples are provided to help add clarity.

2. **Why you may be seeing this expression**

    a. Includes the top reasons I've seen these expressions take place throughout my years of assessing and working with individuals who have an impairment.

3. **Varying responses or interventions for the expression you are seeing**

    a. General interventions are listed. Remember, these need to be customized to your loved one. You will not be able to use them exactly as stated; you will need to generalize these suggestions or statements to suit your loved one. Apply a filter to these as you read them.

    b. Some of these responses or interventions will be for you to complete more observation or assessment. Do not get frustrated, but instead build your understanding of what you are seeing.

— Vocal Expressions —

Vocal expressions can present in many forms. Residents may yell out, appear to be very involved in their thoughts without regard to others, be relatively quiet or isolative regarding verbal speech, or have poor social skills, appearing rude or hurting other's feelings.

- Verbal Outbursts
- Perseveration
- Decreased Conversation Abilities
- Cursing
- Crying Out
- Annoying or Criticizing Others.

 Why these expressions may be taking place:

1. Loss of feelings of control in their life
2. Difficulty processing sensory information
3. Delayed processing speed
4. Pain or discomfort
5. Unmet needs
6. Startle response
7. Loss of filter and ability to put oneself in others' shoes.

Things to Try – "If you are trying, you are succeeding":

- Remain calm. Do not react. Take a deep breath and collect yourself before intervening.
- Validate the individual's feelings—however the person appears to be feeling, state that and let the individual know he or she is justified in this feeling.
- Wait and provide time for a person to answer or interact if the individual has slow processing speed.

- Observe/assess sensory environment. Could the person be over- or under-stimulated? If overstimulated, take the individual to a calm place or reduce stimulation in the current environment. If under-stimulated, provide organized, controlled stimulation to awaken senses.

- Observe/assess for anything that may be creating a startle in the environment. Sit and experience the person's environment. Is there a startling or sudden noise? If so, possibly use a sound machine to eliminate any sudden noises.

- Use patience, acceptance, and love when dealing with a loss of the verbal filter. If a person truly does not understand how he or she may be hurting someone with words, you can't necessarily "fix it." Use distraction and then redirection to take the person's brain off the topic and move it onto something else.

— Aggression —·

The term aggression often gets overused in the world of memory care. Due to the difficulty with communication between affected individuals and their care-givers, misunderstandings frequently happen, leading to "aggressive outbursts." Remaining calm and getting to the root cause to lessen a person's feeling of be-ing threatened is vital. It is essential to use a gentle and calm approach, even if your heart beats out of your chest.

- Threatening Speech or Actions
- Physical Affections
- Aggressive Expressions.

 ## **Why** these expressions may be taking place:

1. Feeling fearful
2. Afraid of caregiver
3. Pain or discomfort
4. Unmet need
5. Feeling rushed
6. Unrealistic expectations—expecting too little and making the person feel like a baby, or expecting too much and creating a feeling of being overwhelmed
7. Verbalizing need for social interaction/touch
8. Feeling of loss of control
9. Misinterpretation of caregiver assistance
10. Reaction to a startle response.

Things to Try – "If you are trying, you are succeeding":

- Remain calm. Do not react. Take a deep breath and collect yourself be-fore intervening.
- Validate individuals' feelings—however they appear to be feeling, state that and let them know they are "justified" in how they feel.
- Wait and provide time for people to answer or interact if they have slow processing speed. Do not rush.

- Offer a hug, handshake, or appropriate touch in place of inappropriate contact.

- Observe/assess sensory environment—could individuals be over or under-stimulated? If overstimulated, take them to a calm place or reduce stimulation in the current environment. If under-stimulated, provide organized, controlled stimulation to awaken senses.

- Observe/assess for anything that may be creating a startle in the environment—sit and experience the environment. Is there a startling or sudden noise? If so, apologize and make the person feel safe. You need to eliminate the fight/flight response he or she feels from being startled.

- Keep other persons safe—if a loved one is becoming physically aggressive and you are unsuccessful in deescalating the moment, move the individual to a new environment. If you're unable to do that, move all other persons to a location where they can be away from the "action." Then go back to the aggressive person to keep him or her safe.

- DO NOT crowd individuals with excess caregivers. This will exaggerate or worsen their symptoms because they will feel threatened (and it heightens the flight/fight response).

— Inappropriate Sexual Expressions —

Sexual expressions are a part of human nature. However, as a person's brain begins to lose the ability to process information the same way it used to, sometimes these expressions can present as "behaviors." Clothing can become overstimulating for people and trigger sexual feelings. People may also speak what is in their head without filtering it first; they may even talk sexually to others or meet their own sexual needs in public places.

- Undressing in Public
- Sexual Innuendos
- Lewd or Rude Remarks
- Masturbation in Public.

 ## **Why** these expressions may be taking place:

1. Uncomfortable clothing
2. Hot/cold
3. Pain or discomfort
4. Unmet need
5. Loss of filter, leading to speaking thoughts
6. Loss of ability to put oneself in others' shoes.

 ## **Things to Try** – "If you are trying, you are succeeding":

- Remain calm. Do not react. Take a deep breath and collect yourself before intervening.
- Meet unmet needs—toileting, incontinence, itchy skin, hot/cold body temperature.
- Try more loose-fitting clothing if tighter clothing is overstimulating.
- Try tighter clothing if loose-fitting clothing is creating sensory defensiveness.

- Distract the individual to take his or her brain off current thoughts—use something that is not related to anything sexual, then redirect to an activity of interest or reminisce about something meaningful to the person.

- Have a frank conversation (do not make the person feel embarrassed or reprimanded) about where it is/is not okay to masturbate. Set up specific times/places that the person can do that successfully and appropriately.

- Never reprimand or scold—distraction is always better.

— Physical Expressions —

Many "physical expressions" are a person's way of adapting to changes in the way the brain processes information. The outward appearance of a behavioral expression, especially when speaking about physical expressions, is often misleading. Trial and error, with multiple adaptations and modifications to the environment, is necessary.

- Sundowning
- Wandering/Pacing/Exit Seeking
- Sleeping During Day
- Insomnia
- Resistance to Care
- Restlessness
- Misuse of Common Objects
- Fluctuating Abilities.

 ## **Why** these expressions may be taking place:

1. Loss of mental energy and attempt to cope with the environment
2. Boredom
3. Pain or discomfort
4. Unmet need
5. Lack of stimulation/under-stimulation
6. Feeling a loss of comfort or security and seeking anything that feels "familiar," "safe," "secure."
7. Feeling the need to "go"—looking for purpose.
8. Difficulty processing sensory stimulation
9. Lack of understanding why a caregiver is trying to assist
10. Miscommunication between caregiver and individual with dementia
11. Fatigue
12. Poor understanding of what objects are or what they are used for, yet a strong need to feel busy and purposeful.

<u>Things to Try</u> – "If you are trying, you are succeeding":

- Remain calm. Do not react. Take a deep breath and collect yourself before intervening.

- Use a schedule of the day to prevent over-/under-stimulation—a nice balance between higher- and lower-stimulating activities and engagements on a rotational basis to keep them balanced.

- Follow an individual's "typical" routine based on life history or verbal report—try to stay as close to the person's routine as possible regarding wake, sleep, level of activity, moments of relaxation, familiar items/objects used, etc.

- Use varying levels of cues to do "with" not "for"—have an accurate understanding of the individual's cognitive level and use verbal, visual, and tactile cues (one, two, or all three types) to add "just the right" assistance to care.

- Anticipate and meet the individual's needs (hunger, thirst, toileting, pain, temperature, level of fatigue, etc.).

- Observe/assess sensory environment—could the person be over- or under-stimulated? If overstimulated, take the person to a calm place or reduce stimulation in the current environment. If under-stimulated, provide organized, controlled stimulation to awaken senses.

- Observe/assess for anything that may be creating a startle in the environment—sit and experience the environment. Is there something that could a startling or sudden noise? If so, possibly use a sound machine to eliminate any sudden noises.

- Promote purpose by understanding the person's identity and finding "occupation"/meaning for the individual in his or her day-to-day interactions in the community.

— Psychological Expressions —.

(i.e., depressive, anxiety, paranoia)

The following "behavioral expressions" are psychological or appear that way. An individual with dementia can have a "dual diagnosis" and have an actual psychological condition in addition to dementia. However, it is essential to distinguish between a real psychological symptom versus a behavioral expression. Use non-pharmacological interventions whenever possible but execute medication when needed.

- Memory Deficit
- Hallucinations
- Delusional Expressions
- Negativism
- Minimal Responses/Withdrawal
- Low Tolerance for Contact
- Irritability
- Adjustment Difficulties
- Social Reluctance
- Paranoid Expressions.

 ## **Why** these expressions may be taking place:

1. Lack of short-term and working memory
2. Visual deficits playing tricks on the individual
3. Hearing deficits playing tricks on the individual
4. Difficulty problem-solving or processing environment or stimulation
5. Vivid dreams or thoughts and limited ability to distinguish reality
6. Inability to use abstract thinking
7. Feeling of loss of control
8. Overstimulation
9. Sensory processing difficulties
10. Fear of the unknown
11. Protective mechanism to keep oneself safe.

<u>Things to Try</u> – "<u>If you are trying, you are succeeding</u>":

- Remain calm. Do not react. Take a deep breath and collect yourself before intervening.

- Validate individuals' feelings—however they appear to be feeling, state that and let them know they are justified in how they feel, even if you must pretend to see/hear what they are expressing. THEY ARE ALWAYS CORRECT in THEIR REALITY.

- Avoid statements like "it's okay" if individuals are upset—something is not okay, so don't try to fix the issue by telling them it is. Validation is much more effective.

- After you have validated an individual's feelings, pretend to "fix" the problem if the hallucination or delusional thought is causing distress.

    Example: If a person is angry at another caregiver for a perceived injustice, a second caregiver can come "be the hero," kick the other person out, and then be the individual's friend to help calm him or her down in that situation.

- Avoid statements like "do you remember me?" or "don't you remember?" or "yesterday, remember we did"—this forces people to use their memory and makes them feel bad, which can create behavioral outbursts, isolation, or withdrawal.

- Observe/assess sensory environment—could the person be over- or under-stimulated? If overstimulated, take the individual to a calm place or reduce stimulation in the current environment. If under-stimulated, provide organized, controlled stimulation to awaken senses.

- Observe/assess for anything that may be creating a startle in the environment—sit and experience the environment. Is there something startling? If so, change your approach or the setting to eliminate this startle.

- Follow an individual's "typical" routine based on life history or verbal report. Try to stay as close to the person's routine as possible regarding wake, sleep, level of activity, moments of relaxation, familiar items/objects used, etc.

- Remain happy, encouraging, and reassuring. Paint a beautiful, descriptive picture to encourage interaction.

- Start conversations and social interactions between two individuals with dementia to help build relationships—dig deep into who the individuals are as people. Avoid questions that require them to talk; instead, you do most of the talking to foster a relationship.

Checklist in Managing What Appear to be "Psych" symptoms – Delusions, Hallucinations, Paranoia...

1. Slow down. Try to listen with your whole self to what your loved one is experiencing. Engage with your loved one to draw out more information and get to the person's reality. This will help you better navigate the symptoms you are seeing. Prevent yourself from reacting out of fear.

2. Be a detective and investigate.

   a. If you are in the home, caring for your loved one alone, you may need to pull in friends or family to investigate and see things from another angle. It isn't easy to see the forest through the trees when you are standing in the middle.

   b. If you are in a skilled care community, hold care huddles with staff. Gather all staff together. Involve the family and friends of the person with dementia. Discuss what you are seeing and brainstorm possible causes with solutions.

3. Journal/log symptoms over time—try not to overreact too quickly. Time is your friend and will help you view multiple similar situations over a period. You may be tempted to place your feelings toward these symptoms onto your loved one. Fight this urge and only observe the person's feelings and thoughts. Use empathy to understand the individual's emotions, rather than inserting your feelings.

4. Go to the person's reality. Put yourself in the individual's shoes. Apply his or her cognitive deficits, sensory deficits, and aging factors. Then try to see if you can understand how there may have been a misperception.

5. Audit the person's world:

   a. Living Environment – light, sound, temperature, routine.

   b. Interpersonal Interaction – how care partners are approaching, interacting, engaging, and relating to the individual.

   c. Medical Information – medications, medical exams, labs.

   d. Changing Factors – even if you think "this can't possibly affect that," pay attention to even subtle changes in your loved one, routines, environment, etc.

6. Reserve medication use for acute delirium or those signs/symptoms that can cause significant harm to the individual or others in the care environment. Work with skilled professionals to help identify when such medications may need to be implemented.

— Mealtime Expressions —·

Mealtime and intake become a topic of conversation as a person progresses through stages of dementia. Often meals become unappetizing; taste buds even may change, making food truly taste differently. Visual deficits can make place settings and multiple options on a table overwhelming and cause an aversion to mealtime. Missing regular oral care can cause buildup in a person's mouth, creating a feeling of "I just ate," thus making the individual want to skip more meals.

- Weight Loss
- Interrupting Others
- Hiding or Hoarding Food
- Slow Eating
- Decision-Making Difficulties.

 ## **Why** these expressions may be taking place:

1. Insufficient intake
2. Lack of adequate oral care
3. Difficulty understanding or using utensils
4. Difficulty processing choices at mealtime
5. Difficulty problem-solving feelings of hunger/fullness
6. Problem processing abstract thinking and needing limited choices
7. Difficulty putting oneself in others' shoes
8. Sensory processing deficit, leading to misinterpretation of food or aversions to certain foods.

 ## **Things to Try** – "If you are trying, you are succeeding":

- Remain calm. Do not react. Take a deep breath and collect yourself before intervening.
- Understand each individual's likes and dislikes and anticipate needs related to mealtime.
- Sit with the individual or individuals at meals to help foster appropriate conversation.

- Sit with the individual to demonstrate the use of utensils and the process of feeding oneself.

- Give the individual enough time for the meal and allow for slow processing. You may need to reheat food halfway through the meal to improve intake.

- Offer six small snacks/meals rather than three large meals; decreasing portion size and increasing frequency can help with intake.

- Offer concrete choices with descriptive words, pictures, visual objects, or two options that get a mutually beneficial answer.

- Use varying levels of cues to do "with" not "for"—have an accurate understanding of the individual's cognitive level and use verbal, visual, and tactile cues (one, two, or all three types) to add "just the right" assistance to care.

- Never reprimand someone for hoarding or taking food; instead, allow it and use distraction or a "trade" of the item for something else later on.

(This list of behavioral expressions is not all-inclusive. Additional training can be obtained from Sarah Viola.)

Appendix B:

RECOMMENDED RESOURCES

The following list contains resources that I have found helpful to guide and inspire my work as an occupational therapist dedicated to helping those living with dementia and their care partners.

Dementia Reconsidered, The Person Comes First by Tom Kitwood

This reading provides an excellent background for why care partners need to apply person-centered care. Professor Kitwood is widely attributed to the development of person-centered care. His definition of humans' psychological needs and extensive research, which provides examples of real-life individuals he studied, gives a great background to why this information is essential to learn and apply.

Dementia Beyond Drugs, Changing the Culture of Care by Dr. Al Power

This reading provides the reader with a shift in thinking, taking a traditionally negative view of those living with dementia and the care provided and turning it into a more positive perspective. Dr. Power offers excellent insight into why the culture of dementia care needed to take a shift in years past. The change in the culture of care has begun, however much work is yet to do if we want to see excellence for those living with dementia. Dr. Power's material can help any care partner shift their thinking and find their foundational "why" for the effort they exert daily to create a higher quality of life for those living with dementia.

Activity Planning Book, How to provide a therapeutic ADL and leisure activity program for persons with dementia by Kim Worchol, OTR/L; Caroline Copeland, OTR/L; and Chris Ebell, OTR/L.

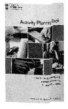
This book provides excellent examples of the varying abilities within cognitive levels as a person progresses through the stages of dementia. It provides detailed descriptions of how to grade or modify activities to an individual's cognitive level to support performance. The ability to perform in meaningful daily tasks and activities shifts as a person progresses in stages of dementia. This material helps the care partner understand what adaptations need to be made to allow the individual living with dementia to continue to participate in varying capacities throughout their progression.

WANT TO TALK TO THE EXPERTS?

For more in-depth Educational & Clinical Needs, Brain Intercept is available to help you assess your loved ones cognitive impairment and provide solutions to help meet your families needs.

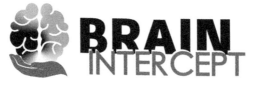

405 8th Ave NW, Suite 203
Aberdeen, SD 57401

(605) 725-8885

BrainIntercept.com
info@brainintercept.com

Sarah Viola & Dr. Harvey Hart co-own a collaborative clinic specifically serving individuals with cognitive impairment and dementia.

Together they opened the clinic to provide early intervention targeting diagnosis, treatment, and ongoing support for persons with cognitive dysfunction and for their care providers.

Dr. Hart named the clinic **Brain Intercept;** intercepting cognitive changes as soon as possible. Early intervention maximizes treatment outcomes and can slow or even stop progression of the disease.

The clinic is a special interest for Dr. Hart after he cared for his late wife who lived with Early Onset Alzheimer's.

"From the mind and heart of a deeply committed professional with a lifelong passion to support families with simple measures to comfort their loved one with dementia and experience the personal joy to the journey's end. The final years with my wife, Velna, carried a mixture of joy alongside pain and grief as dementia eventually took her from us. Ever-Present Insight delivers hope to everyone touched by impaired brain function and brings powerful tools to both professional and personal care providers at all levels of dementia care. The material provides so much help in a small package that would have eased my personal journey."

— Harvey

Made in the USA
Las Vegas, NV
16 January 2022

41407919R00063